4/05

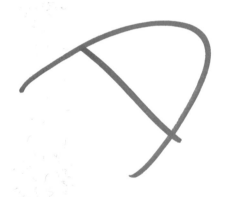

Rescuing
Your Teenager
from Depression

Rescuing
Your Teenager
from
Depression

Norman T. Berlinger, M.D., Ph.D.

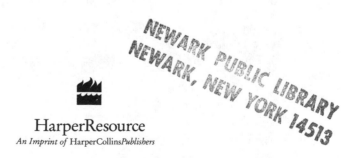

HarperResource

An Imprint of HarperCollinsPublishers

FIRST EDITION

Designed by Joy O'Meara

Library of Congress Cataloging-in-Publication Data

Berlinger, Norman T.
  Rescuing your teenager from depression / Norman T. Berlinger.— 1st ed.
    p. cm.
  Includes index.
  ISBN 0-06-056720-1
    1. Depression in adolescence—Popular works. 2. Parent and teenager. I. Title.

RJ506.D4B476 2005
616.85'27'00835—dc22   2004054368

05 06 07 08 09 WBC/RRD 10 9 8 7 6 5 4 3 2 1

To my son.
He has made me wiser with his struggle.
He has made me braver with his energy and successes.

Contents

Contents

Part 3: *Stay the Watch—Recovery, Recurrences,
and Building Resilience*

Acknowledgments

This book would have been impossible had not so many parents of depressed teens unashamedly stepped forward to tell of their insights, sorrows, and victories.

My son, forever of a generous heart, encouraged me to include his story in this book so that others might benefit from reading about his difficult journey.

The late Conrad Vachon, a distinguished and beloved English teacher at Notre Dame High School in Harper Woods, Michigan, was the first to convince me and many other of his students that the written word is a powerful medium, and that good writing is born of lots of reading (especially the essays of E. B. White). The talented and dedicated faculty at Northwestern University's Medill School of Journalism taught me how to be succinct and how to avoid "word salads." When I was a new reporter at the Minneapolis *StarTribune,* Steve Marcus, the newspaper's science and medicine editor, encouraged me to pursue a writing career. Coming from someone with such a vast experience and such a precise ear for language, his words lit the fire of enthusiasm and provided the major impetus for undertaking this book. I am indeed fortunate to count him as a colleague and friend. Faith Hamlin, my agent at Sanford J. Greenburger Associates, wisely guided this book to the desk of HarperCollins editor Toni Sciarra, whose keen eye resulted in a much improved manuscript. I have learned much about writing from her. Anita W. Bell provided experienced editorial assistance and valuable encouragement when the task sometimes seemed too big.

This book is designed to give information on various medical conditions, treatments, and procedures for your personal knowledge and to help you be a more informed consumer of medical and health services. It is not intended to be complete or exhaustive, nor is it a substitute for the advice of your physician. You should seek medical care promptly for any specific medical condition or problem your child may have. Under no circumstances should medication of any kind be administered to your child without first checking with your physician.

All efforts have been made to ensure the accuracy of the information contained in this book as of the date published. The author and the publisher expressly disclaim responsibility for any adverse effects arising from the use or application of the information contained herein.

The names and identifying characteristics of parents and children featured throughout this book have been changed to protect their privacy.

Before You Begin This Book

This book is about one of the biggest medical impostors I know—teen depression. A depressed teenager may not at all look like the melancholy or moping depressed adult who is your coworker, neighbor, or friend. Instead, you may see anger, hostility, rage, distraction, indifference, procrastination, rebellion, defiance, intoxication, or malaise. A depressed teen may look anything but sad. I learned that as a medical student, and I was reminded when my own son became depressed during his second year of high school.

As parents, we have little difficulty figuring out if our children have chicken pox or tonsillitis. We can even be on the mark when we suspect a bad appendix. But we seem to have big trouble figuring out when their "mood problem" is something more serious than just being cranky, uncooperative, or down in the dumps. Even though we may be guilty of hurrying our children into adulthood, teenagers do not suddenly morph into sophisticated adults. They may not wear their emotions correctly, and we should not take their disposition at face value. Making matters worse, doctors themselves admit that they have not been astute in diagnosing when our children might be depressed. Physicians now calculate that most teen depression goes unrecognized and untreated. The results can be catastrophic.

This book is about wisdom—parents' wisdom. If you want to know something really accurate about yourself, a revealing insight or even a harsh truth, be sure to ask your mother or father. You are just as eagle-eyed about your own children. No one else is. That is why, for this book, I conducted about one hundred interviews of parents who have depressed teenagers. I asked these parents how they figured out the depression, the steps they took to help their children, even how they kept a suicide watch. You will read what worked and what failed. Parents' wisdom comes from the trenches. In every chapter, you will hear their words—what they have to say about emotional health, anger, illicit drugs, intimacy, community, forgiveness, spirituality, therapists, exercise, herbs, the ideal home, high school, college, and how to talk to a teen. As a result, this book is not antiseptically clinical. Yes, all the pertinent medical facts are here. But above all, this book is humanistic, because parents tell how their teen's illness unfolded in their own homes.

This book celebrates the parent. When a child is threatened by an illness, I know of no person who rises up so quickly to the call as a parent, even when tired, troubled, or worried about a stack of overdue bills. I know of no one who joins the battle so tenaciously, or who can so effectively deflate the stigma in which depression seeks its protection. Most of all, a parent owns the crucial ingredient of the prescription against depression—love. There is new and compelling scientific evidence that parents are a vast and invaluable resource in their children's fight against several emotional illnesses, including depression. The misfortune is that this plain fact has not been realized sooner.

The urgent message here is that you should take action. In fact, you may have no choice but to answer the call to become a partnering parent, because your health insurance may limit your teen's access to professional mental health resources. In these pages you will learn the Ten Strategies of Parental Partnering, all derived from parents' experiences, on how to partner with your teen's physician to get the best and quickest results, and to prevent a relapse of the depression. Because I am a physician, I could refine and polish the strategies when necessary.

This is also an optimistic book. Your child's depression is conquerable, and it becomes an especially feeble adversary when a parent is involved in the fight. Moreover, these parents say, when the misery of depression strikes, new bonds, new love, and new insights and skills may be forged from the fire.

In this book, I will ask you to partner with professionals and to closely monitor the life and health of your child. You want to support your teen, but you don't want to intrude. You want to show your concern, but not come off as autocratic. You're probably worried about crossing that mythical dividing line that separates the lives of teens from the lives of parents. You might still hold to the idea that some kind of familial highway exists with teens going one way and parents the other. Veer over the yellow line, and you are guaranteed a head-on collision.

The separateness of teens and parents is a bit of nonsense legitimized for a while by a deplorable notion called the generation gap. Probably because my parents never subscribed to it, neither did I. For several decades, though, I heard it invoked as an easy and ready excuse for all kinds of failures at cooperation or dialogue. The failures most often were due to being closed-minded, not to a chronological difference of twenty-five years. I am most thankful now that that awful notion is being discarded, rightfully tossed into the Dumpster of outmoded or false ideas.

There are several reasons for this happy evolution. One is that baby boomers, who bragged about being alienated from their parents in the sixties, are no longer convinced, as parents themselves, that alienation is such a cool idea. Another is that nowadays parents work especially hard to get involved in their children's lives. Soccer moms are not just a voting bloc. They represent a mind-set among today's mothers and fathers that parents are more than mere chauffeurs and bankrollers. They are cheerleaders, promoters, organizers, publicity agents, mentors, confidants, and counselors. Lastly is the profound and underestimated influence of cell phones and e-mail. When it is so easy to stay connected, it is easy to communicate well and avoid generating chasms of misunderstanding.

And (wow!) teens share this refreshing viewpoint. Recently, national newspapers such as the *New York Times* have reported that high school teachers often hear their students speaking about their parents with warmth, affection, and admiration. College professors hear the same. You have no reason to be intimidated by the generation gap, because it has already been demoted to the dustbin. You also have nothing to fear from that yellow dividing line. It has been replaced by a wide center-lane that you and your teen can travel down together.

There is probably not a moment to spare, because depression is such a painful and debilitating illness. If you suspect your teen might be suffering from depression, read chapters 3 to 5 and learn how to spot the demon. If your teen has already been diagnosed with depression, you are likely becoming aware how scant are the professional resources for combating the illness. Read chapters 6 to 12 and learn how you as a parent can partner with the professionals to speed the recovery along. If your teenager is emerging from depression, read chapters 13 to 14 and learn what good, or treacherous, things might lie on the other side.

Part 1

The Critical Role
of
Parents

1

Escape from the Edge

Eric is fine now.

He is a junior at college majoring in chemistry. I am pleased he no longer isolates himself, and he is adjusting reasonably well to dormitory life with three roommates. In fact, he became the pipe organist for the campus church during his freshman year, playing for Sunday-evening liturgies in front of an audience of seven hundred students, and sometimes bravely conducting the choir even though he had no previous experience. He involves himself in campus life, although I think he could still do better. And he now has enough confidence in his own worth to actively seek out friends and risk the rejection we all fear, instead of waiting for people to come to him.

His sense of humor has returned. The engaging smile that used to spread across his face at the slightest provocation is back as wide as ever. He tells jokes again, and it is good to hear his contagious belly-laugh. He has reclaimed his optimism, too, and he is looking forward to a chemistry internship at a major corporation here in Minnesota this summer. And he can't wait to take those last few flying lessons in order to qualify for his pilot's license. I used to discourage his flying. I worried that the remnants of the depression or the anxiety might interfere with his concentration or his judgment. Now I just have the normal worries about a dear and precious son piloting a flimsy single-engine contraption a mile up in the sky. Eric thoroughly enjoys the hands-on science of flying and says that flying also is a "spiritual experience." As an ever-protective parent, I always remind Eric that for his mother and me it is a spiritual experience, too, but not of the kind he means.

His relationship with his mother, my wife, Pat, is healing quickly, and they are fast friends again. They've picked up where they left off six years ago, and I don't think I see any scars. To see them now, their stormy past relationship, with all the bickering and arguments and sadness, seems incomprehensible. During the time of Eric's most severe depression, Pat worried, and cried, that they would never be close again. But they stay in daily touch now, even when Eric's away at school. Sometimes it's only small talk or a comparison of weather forecasts, but Eric is reminded every day that the distance does not decrease his importance in this family. The cell phone bills are eye-popping, but worth it.

Despite his gratifying comeback from his depression in high school, Eric is not yet on automatic pilot. And so, I must stay closely involved. Certainly, depression has fast-forwarded his development in areas such as emotional maturity, problem solving, and empathy. But he seems a bit behind on assertiveness and self-reliance, because teen depression is a disease of emotional detours. While his high school classmates were thinking about colleges or careers, Eric was desperately trying to find a reason to get out of bed in the morning.

While other teens were piling up confidence, Eric was searching for reasons not to hate himself. And while other teens were joining clubs and building relationships, Eric was isolating himself in his room and watching movies, sometimes the same movie over and over as if in a trance. Depression didn't make Eric a coward, but it paralyzed him with its pain.

The course has not been smooth, but it has been steady.

I needed to stay closely involved when Eric left for college to help him catch up from the detours. Eric did not become the pipe organist by accident. I "engineered" that by approaching the church's music director to take him on, only because Eric had not yet regained the self-esteem to do it alone. And I "arranged" for Eric's freshman residence hall to be a special "first-year experience": three hundred incoming freshman gathered into one dormitory as a nurturing community in order to smooth the adjustment to parent-free college life and to facilitate making friends. Every so often I search my soul to make sure I am being truly helpful rather than overly protective or meddlesome. It doesn't take long to remember that the depression so completely ravaged Eric's energy, optimism, and sense of worth that I must not be merely his sideline coach, but his side-by-side teammate. I cannot just stand behind the bench, encouraging him on. I must be on the treacherous field of play with him. I'm convinced now that anything less is a grievous error. So, too, is William Styron. In a poignant account of his own depression, he says, "Calling 'chin up' from the safety of the shore to a drowning person is tantamount to insult."

The Transformation

Eric was fine six years ago, too, a model fourteen-year-old. And I was unaware of the peril ahead.

Parents who met him often told me they wanted a child just like him. He was charming, polite, and humorous. Most of all, Eric was kind. As a high school freshman, his teachers acknowledged him in a class assembly as the most congenial and helpful student there. They awarded him a framed certificate, which I recently found in one of his drawers and put out for display again in his room. Looking at that certificate brings back all the wrenching memories, because that award marks the beginning of his downhill slide into the darkness.

Eric's nightmare in his last three years of high school became my nightmare, too. His personality deteriorated, and the Eric I knew was slipping away at a terrifying speed. His mood turned sour, and he became belligerent, but usually only with his mother. A vicious stranger seemed to have moved into Eric's body, and he argued about anything important to the family—doing homework, attending tennis practice, or what time to set for a reasonable evening curfew. His arguing was no less passionate about inconsequential things, such as whether his mother was littering the car floor with sesame seeds from her eat-while-driving breakfast. Eric would pick a fight, stay on the attack, and not back off until his mother was in tears. I still wonder why I was often spared.

His sense of self-worth crashed, and afraid of people, he gradually stopped asking friends over to our house. The first hint of the crash was his fifteenth birthday party. I found it peculiar that he relinquished some of his thunder by inviting a classmate whose birthday was the same week to have a "coparty" at our house. Eric didn't believe in himself any longer, and I didn't realize this was Eric's strategy to make sure his party wasn't a Stella Dallas kind of flop. Soon after, he was isolating himself in his room. The pathological inwardness that is one of depression's demons forced Eric to erect around himself an impenetrable cell of solitary confinement.

Studying became as difficult as mingling with people. At the beginning of his sophomore year, Eric surprised me with a nightly request to help him with his geometry homework even though he had a knack for math. Later he would tell me, "Studying was scary because I was alone with myself." As the depression deepened, he lost his ability to concentrate. "I would read the same sentence over and over and never get it," he said. Overwhelmed, he gave up. "Who cares about school when you think everyone hates you?" he said. Thus the suffocating cloak of depression's pessimism enveloped him.

His energy crashed, too. He quit being the piano accompanist for school musical events. He withdrew from extracurricular activities. It was a chore to get him to tennis practice. At tennis meets or tournaments he would play with unabashed indifference. The best he could do was go through the motions of living. He had become an automaton.

Eric had gotten the gift of gab from his mother, a warm and engaging woman who can make you feel as if you have known her for a long time after talking with her for only a few minutes. But Eric's facility with speech evaporated during the depression. "I was picking the wrong words," he said. "I was even slurring my words like I had been drinking alcohol." Soon, Eric was at a loss for words. He would answer questions with terse replies, or he would pepper his language with filler phrases, like "sounds good to me," to disguise his conversation as lively and responsive. Eric's mind couldn't think of anything to say.

Eric wasn't just withering. He took on new and sometimes peculiar personality traits that said for sure he was undergoing a transformation.

Like most depressed teens, Eric desperately sought an antidote for what he thought was sadness. He pursued nonstop entertainment: car stereos, DVD movies, and flight-simulation software occupied most of his time after school instead of homework. Once he got his driver's license, he added new amusements—downtown dance clubs (admission gained with a phony ID) or aimless cruising. The amusements didn't improve his mood. They merely distracted him from the mysterious and intensely uncomfortable emotions inside him. And all the activity never generated friendships. "I didn't want friends," Eric said. "I wanted acquaintances. It was too much work to have friends. I was afraid to work for their approval."

I had never figured out that Eric was using coffee as another antidote. The depression had so squelched Eric's spontaneity that he used caffeine to undo the "mental blockage." On his way to school he always stopped at Caribou Coffee, Minneapolis's equivalent of Starbucks, for a big morning dose. "That was why I was usually twenty or thirty minutes late for school. But I always made such good excuses that I only got two detentions. I was 'normally' depressed with coffee, but terribly depressed without it. You know, Dad, depressed people need a mental wheelchair." I used to chide him then that all that coffee made him jittery and unattractive. Only later did I understand that he had a compelling reason to suffer caffeine's adverse effects.

Eric's sleeping patterns turned bizarre. He would lie awake in the dark confessional of an insomniac night and examine every piece of evidence he could find to justify his self-loathing. Soon, he was stuffing his medicine cabinet with bottles of over-the-counter sleeping remedies or antihistamines that warned of the side effect of drowsiness. I didn't know until later that he often drank himself to sleep and in the morning was sneaking out the empty beer cans in his school backpack. Although the nighttime wakefulness was exquisitely painful, sometimes he would prevent himself from falling asleep to gain a peculiar advantage for the next day. "Being tired in the morning let me be more spontaneous at school because the grogginess broke down the defenses," Eric said. Then he would "dose up" on coffee to allow out what was left of his personality. Eric was sleepless at night and exhausted during the day. I'm sure the combination was torture.

Eric abandoned his old friends. He no longer felt worthy of their friendship, and he was afraid they would be turned off by his depression if discovered. But Eric wanted to put on a show at school that he wasn't a loner, so he picked up a collection of new friends. "I was a great friend to the exchange students," he said. "Even though they speak good English, they are still 'outside' and want to have someone to talk to. Gay kids make good friends, too. They are going through their own kind of hell in high school and are not judgmental of you if they figure out you're depressed. The worst guys I hung around with were the guys who chewed tobacco. We had a 'club' because we were passing around a tin in the lavatory or in the back of the classroom. They didn't ask any questions. They didn't care."

A Mystery

For teenagers, depression is a mental wilderness. Eric couldn't figure out what was wrong.

My wife and I hadn't yet figured it out, either. I was focusing on the consequences of Eric's problem rather than on the problem itself. I am still surprised I missed this one for so long.

After all, I was a physician, and a good one, too, I thought. I had graduated from the University of Michigan Medical School in Ann Arbor, a remarkable and enlightened institution that made sure every doctor-to-be studied adult and child psychiatry each year of the four-year curriculum. As a senior-year research project, I worked with the student health-service psychiatrists who wanted to investigate the eventual academic success of undergraduate students who required hospitalization for emotional illness. My research was good enough that I was invited to present the results at a national meeting of the American Psychiatric Association. I even worked evenings at a mental health crisis clinic. Once in practice, it didn't take long to realize that much of the illness I was seeing in my patients was actually stress or depression, purely so, or combined with their physical ailments. I knew when my patients' psyches needed medical care. I thought I was quite astute.

Still, I had forgotten the adage about how depression often manifests itself in teenagers: bad or mad may actually mean sad.

In fact, my realization that Eric was depressed was more an intuition than a conscious and calculated diagnosis. One evening while my wife and I were arguing about Eric's obnoxious behavior in front of him, I suddenly blurted out to her, "Damn it. Can't you see he's depressed?" Then came a long and unexpected silence in the room while the three of us tried to figure out what had just transpired. My wife resumed the conversation and vehemently dismissed the possibility. After all, depression could mean that we had failed Eric as parents, and egregiously so. Eric stared at me with a bit of surprise and, of all things, hope, because he was considering that I had stumbled onto the explanation for the dark mystery inside him. And I was carefully reconsidering what I had just said to make sure it was accurate.

I was forced to figure this one out myself, because no one else was helpful.

None of Eric's teachers had a clue about his depression. After all, school was Eric's main stage, as it is for any teenager, and he cleverly disguised it there. While I was interviewing Eric for this book, he told me that his junior-year journalism teacher was once worried enough about him to refer him to a school counselor. "I blew them both off, and that was the end of it," Eric said. Neither of them ever phoned us to voice their concerns.

None of Eric's friends approached me to say that Eric was

worried, and at times even frantic and hyperactive. It's no surprise. Teenagers usually avoid discussing uncomfortable topics such as emotional health with adults. In fact, it wasn't until recently that the mother of one of Eric's high school friends told me, "Peter knew all along that Eric was struggling."

None of my friends, especially the ones who were dealing with their own depressed teens, gave me any hints about what depression looks like in teenagers. These parents allowed the stigma of depression to stifle any conversation about it beyond the fortress of their home. Only later, when I told them I was writing this book, did they think it safe to admit they had had a depressed teenager of their own. In fact, most of these parents asked to be interviewed, especially the mother whose son shot himself last year. Having suffered in self-imposed isolation and silence, they wanted to share their stories, both as a help for other parents and as a catharsis for themselves. I've come to realize that all around us are legions of parents with depressed teens. They are eager, even desperate, to speak, but only when it is safe.

Where to Turn?

Depression is grave mental disease, but I didn't get much help finding a therapist, either.

I'm no longer surprised about that, although my sense of urgency left me frustrated and angry then. Eric needed a therapist specializing in adolescent mental health, and so the morning after my epiphany about Eric's depression, I put in a frantic call to his pediatrician. Dr. S. mechanically recited a list of six therapists, but, remarkably, he didn't voice any preferences. In fact, he didn't even ask to see Eric as a patient to make sure my assessment was correct. As I think back now, none of that should have come as a surprise. After all, Dr. S., like most primary-care physicians, wasn't especially well trained to identify depression.

Then I called Deacon M. at our church, an energetic and nurturing place that tried to address the diverse needs of its congregation. All he could offer was the name of one overworked psychologist whom he considered helpful.

A neighbor down the street, Dr. K., was my last resort. He was a pediatrician who was a model for other physicians on how to care for patients. But the adolescent psychiatrist to whom he referred me was too booked up to see Eric, and she suggested a therapist whom she respected.

Eric was in pain, but the adolescent psychiatrists on Dr. S.'s list all were too busy to see him for several months. More of these doctors are leaving practice than entering it in Minnesota, and this is a national trend. In fact, the average age of an adolescent psychiatrist in Minnesota is sixty-two. Deacon M.'s recommendation of a psychologist proved less than satisfactory. I made an appointment with her and explained Eric's situation. Without hesitation, she made an unflinching prescription that, for Eric's good, the family ought to be dissolved—and after hearing only what I had to say. Maybe she should have waited to hear what Eric and my wife had to say.

I was now down to the colleague-of-a-colleague-of-a-neighbor. This therapist, Paul L., had an appointment available in six weeks. When I interviewed him, he seemed satisfactory because his goals appeared to be the goals of our family. I entrusted Eric to him.

Entrust is the key word. Like any child, Eric was precious. After thirteen years of infertility, with the gnawing sadness that only infertile couples ever understand, my wife conceived Eric. But she was then thirty-six, categorically a "high-risk pregnancy." It seemed only natural then that Eric would come into the world prematurely, and with respiratory distress syndrome and streptococcal sepsis, newborn diseases with frighteningly high morbidity and mortality rates. Eric struggled for breath and for his life for three weeks. Ultimately he won, ridding himself of the ventilator, chest tubes, and IV infusions of the neonatal intensive care unit. He was long-awaited and hard-won.

A Partner out of Necessity

For depression, there is no easy way out. That is why a depressed person desperately needs a helpmate. I never set out intentionally to be a partner with the medical professionals who treated Eric. It evolved that way out of necessity.

I started out playing a self-assigned smaller role, although it didn't feel right. Eric had to wait at least six weeks to see a therapist. He had to wait just as long for the prescribed antidepressant medication to exert its first beneficial effects. But his suffering was acute every day. How could he muster the energy to get out of bed in the morning? Would he harm himself? How to ease his ordeal in the meantime? For those first six weeks, much of what I did was only to reassure Eric that his medicine would "kick in anytime now," and that his appointment with the therapist was coming up soon. A mere cheerleader, all I was doing was telling Eric, "Chin up." But I concluded I had an emergency on my hands, and if Eric were one of my surgical patients with an infected or dehiscing incision, I would immediately have marshaled the hospital's operating-room personnel and resources to fix the problem, in the middle of the night if necessary. For the immense suffering it causes and for the potential threat to life it poses, it is a serious mistake to view depression as something less urgent.

Then things got worse.

Eric's medicine did finally kick in, but the improvement in his mood was disappointing. Moreover, the antidepressant was making his insomnia worse, a known side effect, and Eric was on the verge of becoming nocturnal. After he spent a few fifty-minute sessions with the therapist, I asked for an appointment also, to check on Eric's progress. The therapist turned out to be well-intentioned, but dangerously off the mark. He was giving Eric generic textbook advice, which, however, was counterproductive for the specific context in which Eric lived. It was also contrary to the goals of our family. Ultimately, the therapist admitted his prejudice that depressed teens ought to be viewed as victims of circumstances rather than as patients with a disease. This position is antiquated and untenable, since most psychiatrists now believe that the combination of both viewpoints yields the most accurate explanation for the illness.

Desperate for help, Eric had joined a support group at his high school, but it wasn't helping either. Although his high school rightfully prides itself as being attentive to its students' emotional health, it does not have the resources to be all things to all people. Like most high schools, its support groups are run by well-meaning but insufficiently trained personnel. In addition, since there was no depression-specific support group at Eric's high school, he joined the "situations" group, composed of sad students who were struggling with impending parental divorce, emerging homosexuality, or an addiction. "They spent most of their time bashing parents," Eric said. He dropped out after several meetings.

Eric was not getting better—and he was becoming desperate for some relief. That's why one evening, in an eerily casual manner, he confided to me, "Now I know why people commit suicide." Later he would tell me, "I didn't have a plan, but I could see myself doing it. I had two of those suicide days. Death seemed nice." Eric was losing hope for deliverance.

Now I was desperate, too.

When a teenager uses the word *suicide,* a parent should never dismiss the remark as anything less than a flashing red alert. I knew

I was helping in those few early months, but I was only a bit player. Now I hunkered down into crisis mode and came out in full force. I would take the reins if I had to. The stakes were too high to do otherwise. Only later did I realize what I had determined to become: a true partner with his therapist. My participation had to be significant, because the resources available were unsatisfactory. I qualified as the best partner because I was his parent. I knew him better than any therapist. I worked from a basis of love and logic. Moreover, I had 24-7 access to Eric.

Depression never allows a quick rescue. There was a lot of work to do. I shifted into high gear.

I devised plans to counteract depression's two main demons—worthlessness and hopelessness. So as not to undermine anyone else's authority, I told Eric I was his "therapist at home." I drew up lists of tasks to accomplish with Eric, such as bolstering his self-esteem or forcing him into a tennis game despite his disinterest, and planned each night which ones would be addressed the next day. Since boys respond well to "instrumental" solutions such as activities and diversions, I planned movies, concerts, a road trip to Chicago, visits to relatives in Detroit, restaurant meals, biking, or just ordinary drives around Lake Minnetonka so we could chat in the car. I even became a mall rat with him on those days when it seemed that just plain hanging out would do some good. More important, I identified the cognitive restructuring tasks that needed attention in order to unwind his "stinky thinking" and would give Eric specific messages and ideas each day as if I were a cognitive therapist. I kept careful track to make sure no item on my task list was missed. I kept an insomnia watch, and I kept a suicide watch.

At times I doubted that I was accomplishing anything substantive. For example, during all the activities I planned with Eric, I never stopped talking so that he would know I was always thinking about him. But, I wondered, was I offering him nothing more than consolation? Last summer, though, when Eric was home from college, he told me, "You helped me because you were always willing to talk about me. You let me vent." The black hole of depression is inwardness. The constant conversation let him escape the hole for a while.

It's easy to doubt your efforts because a depressed person often is incapable of showing the results you want. The depression flattened Eric's emotions, and I often couldn't read whether he was responding to my efforts. Depression also so drained his initiative that sometimes he couldn't implement a solution, even a simple and easy one. Yes, some things may not have done much good then. But never underestimate a teenager. Eric takes into his memory banks everything a parent says. "The talks we had come back to me now," he told me last month. "A lot of them didn't really help then, because there was nothing left to work with. But they help now."

At the time, my best accomplishments were the least obvious. A good deal of what I tried didn't seem to move Eric forward. "But the things you did prevented me from getting worse," he told me later. Many times, I wasn't lifting him from the ledge. But I was providing him a high and sturdy guardrail so he wouldn't tumble off. Hopelessness is one of depression's twin demons, and teenagers, by definition, are immature and often feel powerless to solve big problems. It didn't matter one iota whether I got any positive feedback. I stayed involved every day if only to show him that someone of power had been recruited into his fight.

The crucial ingredient, though, was to provide a strong home.

Our family is definitely not the idyllic Nelsons or Cleavers. Like all real-life families, we have our share of dysfunctions, some of them serious. But Eric could readily see that those dysfunctions were always being addressed. He could see that his family was constantly working to solve its problems and make itself better. That's what makes any family successful, and that's why Eric believed his family was a solid asset on which he could rely. "You have a philosophy that the center must hold," he told me several months ago. "Because of that, my home was a very safe place. I could be myself. I felt great at home. That's why I didn't do drugs when I was depressed. I didn't need any other kind of escape. My home was my escape."

Unfortunately with depression, an escape has a downside. "Home was my hideout," Eric said. "I could isolate myself." At the very time I didn't want Eric isolating himself from friends at school, I was providing an attractive place to enable and reinforce his isolation. I realized it was happening, but I felt that the huge benefits of home's safe harbor and refuge far outweighed that particular disadvantage. I would have to attend to the issue later.

The task of being a parent-partner during Eric's depression was immensely tiring, sometimes exhausting. After all, it was another job. To educate myself about teen depression required a lot of reading and studying to draw up a list of "prescriptives" that was on the mark for Eric, and it took a lot of time to implement them. It also required heavy doses of meditation, soul-searching, and prayer.

The task was threatening, too. Psychologists have long appreciated that the cause, course, and resolution of teen depression depends a lot on family dynamics. I had to force myself to take inventory of the family and determine where my wife and I might be causing any turmoil that contributed to Eric's depression. Moreover, parsing the turmoil involves ascribing blame, and that causes its own bit of trouble. The family situation gets worse before it gets better. The inventory was an especially difficult task because Eric's mother doubted the depression, and only in the past year has she actually admitted it and used the word *depressed* in reference to him.

I regret my reluctance at the time to talk to other parents with depressed teenagers, and I regret their being ashamed to talk to me. We could have learned effective strategies, forged in the fire, for combating the ogre. No textbook guidelines or generic advice, this stuff, but tested weapons that helped and perhaps even saved their children. Maybe they would have worked for Eric, too. I intend to set them down in this book.

For adults, I think of depression mostly as a disease of emotional detours, and a depressed adult will need to make up for a lot of time lost to inactivity. But for teenagers, I think it also has the potential to be a disease of subtractions if not attended to promptly. It occurs at an especially vulnerable time in their emotional gestation when they are forming fundamental attitudes and their identities. Ignored or poorly treated depression can mutate a teen's psyche as certainly as a toxic chemical will misshape a fetus developing in the womb. These teens will ratchet down their spontaneity and optimism. Or they will forever panic over worries that a few days in a funk means the ogre is reawakening. Worst of all, they might lose confidence in themselves, having never completely recovered from the delirium of worthlessness.

Eric escaped most of that. The adversity introduced Eric to himself, and in many respects now he is mature beyond his years. He is clearly richer in reliable problem-solving strategies. Six years later, he is still making up for lost time, but I think he knows how to sail the big and treacherous waves without sinking.

2

Parents Matter

What would you do if your child had an acute physical illness? Of course, you would take her to the doctor and get her the prescribed medicine. But it's likely that you would want to do more—such as research the illness on the Internet, perhaps go for a second opinion, and make sure she was diligently following all the doctor's suggestions. You would want to monitor the illness closely and do everything in your power to support her recovery.

Depression must be approached by parents with the same earnestness as a severe physical ailment—because depression *is* a genuine illness. It is as genuine as asthma or diabetes, and among teenagers it is just as prevalent. It causes real physical symptoms—insomnia, fatigue, malaise, and weight loss. And it causes pain. The pain is emotional, but that is no consolation. Just ask around. Most people would prefer enduring physical pain rather than emotional pain. Depression requires medicines, and occasionally hospitalization. It is a genuine illness due to the collapse of certain brain functions. And sometimes, depression turns fatal.

Never, never look upon it as a weakness, a character flaw, or a mere state of mind. Outraged at this entrenched and wrongheaded stigmatization, the U.S. surgeon general felt it necessary several years ago to remind us, "There is no scientific reason to differentiate between mental health and other kinds of health. Mental illnesses are physical illnesses."

A serious illness is guaranteed to disrupt a life.

Depression disrupts all the teen's assumptions. I will fall in love. I will always look forward to canoeing. I will live to be twenty-one. The happy assumptions are now replaced by a dark and terrible question: What is going on here?

Depression disrupts your teen's biography and self-concept, because uncertainty looms large in the experience of any serious illness. A teenager is unsure about the impact and the course of the disease. What do I look and sound like? How can I ever get some sleep? How can I keep from hurting myself?

Depression also depletes your teen's resources. Friendships are abandoned. Community involvement withers. Even everyday activities like eating or listening to music are difficult to maintain. Daily life becomes a burden of conscious and deliberate action. The disruptions give a parent a sense of catastrophe. After all, our children are natural innocents, and their futurity is threatened.

From Parent to Caregiver

There is no easy way out of depression. That is why a depressed person desperately needs a helper, a champion who is both supporter and warrior.

In the midst of his own catastrophic depression, William Styron says he was blessed with two. Nearly every day he stayed in touch by telephone with a close friend, a newspaper columnist, whose "support was untiring and priceless. It was he who kept admonishing me that suicide was unacceptable. I still look back on his concern with immense gratitude." And his wife, his mainstay, was "the endlessly patient soul who had become nanny, mommy, comforter, priestess, and most importantly, confidante—a counselor of rocklike centrality to my existence whose wisdom far exceeded that of Dr. Gold. I would hazard the opinion that many disastrous sequels to depression might be averted if the victims received support such as she gave me."

With an ill child in the house, the parent automatically becomes a caregiver. It seems only natural, and a parent even welcomes the opportunity to help ease chicken pox, coach crutch-walking, or administer insulin injections. It may not come as naturally to act as a caregiver when the illness is emotional, but it's just as essential.

Your depressed teenager is not only sick but also disabled. Depression is so toxic to the intellect that it poisons the ability to think, and it destroys initiative. You must step in if only because of the paralysis.

Because depression is an emotional illness, you may wonder whether you're qualified to handle this kind of problem. It ought to be self-evident: no one is better qualified than a parent to be an emotional caregiver, because parents are the most powerful influences on their teenagers' lives.

To write this book, I conducted about one hundred interviews of parents of depressed teens. Their insights about how they positively influenced the course of the depression would provide a long and reassuring litany. I've distilled their comments into a list of the seven unique powers that parents have to help conquer the demon.

The Seven Parental Powers

Parental Power #1—No other person is as sensitive to the development of the teen's interior life as a parent.

Parental Power #2—A parent is the primary generator of a teen's self-esteem. When depression causes its poisonous self-loathing, a parent becomes the most potent soldier in this perverse battle to reclaim self-worth.

Parental Power #3—A parent is the ultimate reality check. Psychologist David Elkind is always ready to correct the modern misconception that teenagers are sophisticated thinkers. By definition, they are immature. Ordinarily, they have difficulty with abstract thinking and limited abilities to formulate problem-solving strategies. Their situation is much worse when they're depressed.

Parental Power #4—A parent is the guardian of the teen's biography. A depressed teenager worries about the permanent impairment the illness will cause, and whether he will survive at all. In the midst of depression, the outcome always appears uncertain.

Parental Power #5—A parent has 24-7 access to the teenager. No one else does. And no one else is always willing to help, if only to be available in the wings for an opinion.

Parental Power #6—A parent is the best person to help the teen pass as normal during the most embarrassing or disabling periods of the depression.

Parental Power #7—Most important, all of a parent's actions, even the ordinary ones, are done out of love. It's no wonder, then, that the sacred is often portrayed as a parent. So great is their love that parents will risk an angry confrontation with their teens, or even vilification, to make sure things go right for them.

Author David Spangler sums it up best in his book *Parent as Mystic, Mystic as Parent*. He says the parent is "the portal through which a human soul becomes part of the world." A depressed teenager is a kidnapped prisoner, and the parent is the only real portal for entry back into the world.

Any serious illness disrupts not only the life of the sufferer, but also the life of the caregiver. The disruption is the price the caregiver pays, and sociologists call it engulfment.

Your everyday life is engulfed. It gets reorganized and starts to revolve around your depressed teen. Your schedule no longer is your own. Prescriptions must be filled, medicines taken, appointments made. You give your teenager comfort and companionship, even if, as an adolescent, she doesn't desire the presence of a parent. And you keep careful watch.

Your personal life is disrupted, too. Because you feel the need to be closer to your depressed teenager, you may increase the distance between you and your other children, and perhaps also between you and your spouse. Guilt, regret, and conflict are the unfortunate by-products. Since the role of parent-as-caregiver is constructed as one of obligation and selflessness, there's a tendency to delegitimize your own needs, and you may pay insufficient attention to yourself. Your own biography suffers—you must make the transition from the parent of a happy and healthy child to the parent of a teenager in crisis. All the while you search for an explanation. How could this happen to my child, to my family? What did I do wrong?

The price is mitigated, though. The parents whom I interviewed for this book uniformly felt that it was a privilege to be allowed the most intimate kind of participation in their teen's interior life. And they became convinced, if not convinced before, that family life, even with its ordeals, is the most precious kind of time.

From Caregiver to Partner

The importance of partnering with a health professional in combating illness is not at all a new idea, but it is just now coming of age.

Partnering goes several important steps beyond caregiving. Rather than merely agreeing to the health professional's prescribed treatment program, the partner assumes a meaningful role in formulating that program. Rather than unswervingly carrying out the health professional's treatment instructions, the partner judges, within set limits, when and how to modify the instructions, if necessary. In the extreme, should the health professional no longer be able to deliver care, the partner takes over as much as legitimately possible. Whatever the degree of the partner's participation, the partner assumes a degree of accountability for the patient's outcome.

One of the first instances of partnering arose almost fifty years ago on America's obstetric wards. Men were no longer mere witnesses to the birth of their children. Obstetricians and midwives recruited them to be their partners on behalf of the mothers. Partnering men orchestrated breathing interventions during labor, cut the cord immediately after delivery, and provided invaluable emotional support throughout. No longer relegated to being buck privates through labor and delivery, they became lieutenants, but always answerable to the generals.

At about the same time, partnering was starting to prove itself as a valuable resource in mental health care. Public policy debates then seriously questioned the validity of chronic institutionalization of adolescent and young-adult schizophrenic patients, with the result that some of the responsibility for care was turned over to the parental home. Parental partnering with psychiatrists in the treatment of their schizophrenic children yielded gratifying results. Parent-managed patients had fewer exacerbations of schizophrenia, less intense schizophrenic symptoms, fewer hospital admissions, and a reduced need for antipsychotic medications. Family-based management was a resounding success.

Although later studies of other emotional illnesses were not as exhaustive, the value of structured parental involvement was affirmed. Parents made a clear and lasting difference in the outcomes for their children with phobias, obsessive-compulsive disorders, drug abuse, conduct disorders, bipolar disorder, and anxiety syndromes. They usually made a big difference in depression, too.

The era of parental indictment has finally come to an end. For a century, parents had suffered from the unsubstantiated notions of psychiatrists and psychologists who considered the family a pathological entity. Over one hundred years ago, one physician, William Gull, claimed that parents were the "worst attendants" for their children with anorexia nervosa. Another physician, Jean-Martin Charcot, sought to suppress the visits of parents to their emotionally ill children because their presence was thought to prevent progress. If parents weren't being viewed as counterproductive, they were often considered unnecessary. It was all wrong, and wrongful, too.

Consumerism has fostered a new mutuality in health care. Patients, and parents of patients, are now wiser, smarter, and more assertive. Accurate and detailed information about health-care quality, treatments, options, and costs is readily available from newspapers, magazines, television, and the Internet. Especially as health-care dollars shrink, parents come to physicians expecting help to achieve outcomes for their children on which they have often already decided—more so if their child's disease appears long-term, such as asthma, diabetes, or depression. Physicians no longer deliver purely physician-decided care. Increasingly, they try to meet consumer-identified needs. If dissatisfied, parents don't hesitate to exercise their option for a second opinion. Physician paternalism is out. Mutuality is in. This mutuality is just beginning to be called partnering. Despite the approaching tidal wave, many health-care providers are still resisting the notion. Many others, though, are receptive.

Psychologists at the University of Pennsylvania and the University of Miami have gone a step further. In their own words, they have ratified the concept of parental partnering in the family-based treatment of teenagers with emotional illnesses as the "therapist-parent alliance." The alliance generates significant spin-offs—parents usually improve communication with their teens, resolve more conflicts, and strengthen their mutual attachment. Parent-teen attachment may sound corny to some, but never underestimate its importance. These same psychologists have shown that stronger attachment leads to significant reductions in the teen's depression. If better attachment is the only benefit of the therapist-parent alliance, it is still huge.

This new therapist-parent alliance concept recently passed a stiff test in the family-based treatment of teenage anorexia nervosa, a severely debilitating disease that is fatal in 6 to 10 percent of adolescents and accompanied by depression in up to 50 percent of them.

Psychiatrists at London's Maudsley Hospital rejected the notion of the pathological family and devised a treatment plan based on large-scale parent participation. They also rejected the flawed notion, popular among some baby boomers, that a teenager ought to be as autonomous as possible and the parent ought to stay on the sidelines and be more of a peer or a pal to the teen. Focusing on the family as a necessary resource for recovery, the Maudsley approach makes parents partners and puts them in charge of feeding their teenager as if she were starving for some other medical reason. In anorexia, food is medicine, and the parents are instructed not to back down. The parents offer the teen incentives to eat, or the family sits at the dinner table, for hours if necessary, until the meal is consumed. In rare circumstances, the parents may resort to spoon-feeding. Simultaneously, the parents work with the teen on the major tasks of adolescence—socialization, sexuality, and independence. One characteristic of teenagers with an emotional illness is that they have difficulty motivating themselves to get better. The involvement of parents gets around this unfortunate tendency, and teens enrolled in the Maudsley method have shown a remarkably high rate of treatment adherence.

When parents get involved as partners and see the process through, the results with the Maudsley approach are impressive in reversing restrictive eating. The outcomes of anorexic teenagers bent on self-starvation are clearly better with family-based treatment than with individual treatment with a psychotherapist. So far, psychiatrists at Stanford University are achieving a success rate of about 90 percent after just six months of family-based treatment for anorexia nervosa. Other studies show that the success is maintained for years. Furthermore, this kind of parental partnering is now proving highly effective for teenagers who binge eat and purge.

The idea of the therapist-parent alliance is now finding its way into the treatment of severely depressed teenagers who have attempted suicide. Psychologist Cheryl King, the director of the Child and Adolescent Depression Program at the University of Michigan, has recently developed a unique social-network intervention program called the Youth Nominated Support Team (YST) to supplement traditional psychiatric treatment. Partnering is its philosophical keystone.

"Teenagers don't get excited about coming in to talk about their emotional health with a strange adult," King says. "So I ask depressed teenagers to nominate four adults from different domains of their life to give them a wide, wraparound support network. About seventy-five percent of them nominate at least one parent. Other nominees are coaches, grandparents, aunts, or uncles. At least twenty percent nominate someone from their religion. I give the parents the veto power over nominations." The healing process is intimate and collaborative.

The four partnering adults receive training, called psycho-education, that focuses on the teenager's psychiatric illness, the individualized treatment plan, suicide risk factors, and the ways of accessing emergency services. The four support persons meet individually, casually and unobserved, with the depressed teenager at least once a week to listen to the teenager's concerns and to solve problems. They make sure the teen is adhering to the treatment plan and also assess whether there is progress toward the treatment goals, or regression into worsening depression or to an increased risk of suicide. All the while, mental health professionals are maintaining regular weekly contact with the partnering adults.

"YST is highly effective at reducing suicidal thoughts and emotional distress," King says, "and these extremely ill teenagers show improved adaptive functioning." She is not yet sure why girls seem to get better results than boys. YST is a work in progress, and the latest information about it can be found on its Web site: www.med .umich.edu/psych/yst.

A Mandate to Be a Partner

An episode of major depression is a calamity for a teenager. Self-esteem plummets, and the teen gathers evidence, even manufacturing it, to justify a merciless self-hatred. A sense of the future evaporates because the unremitting emptiness of the present disallows a vision of a tomorrow. Unable to understand the mystery inside them, teens often act out the mystery, and peculiarly so, with hostility, drug abuse, sexual promiscuity, dangerous risk-taking, or antisocial behavior.

It is no wonder, then, that the prescription of an antidepressant medication so often is an incomplete treatment for a major depression. A small pill from a bottle is powerless to totally counteract all these huge aberrations of thinking. As the aberrations take hold, episodes of major depression often run a chronic course, with the episode stretching out for many months, recurring quickly, or even disallowing a complete remission between episodes.

Without psychotherapy, a teen runs the risk of poisoned thinking, perhaps for years, perhaps for a lifetime. Pills are good and necessary—but they may not be enough. Only recently have mental health professionals scientifically addressed the issue of a combined treatment for serious depression. Studies are now showing that pharmacotherapy and psychotherapy are additive—the sum is greater than the whole. In fact, the combination of both increases the likelihood of a good response to treatment by at least 30 percent. The new science is now supporting the old widespread clinical impression that combined therapy is superior and leads to higher recovery rates and to a shorter time to recovery.

Psychotherapy to help a person think through the depression is especially important for teenagers because their thinking abilities are not yet fully developed. They need all the help they can get in this regard. After all, only around the age of twelve does an adolescent begin the maturational move out of concrete thinking into higher abstract thinking. Teens are only beginning to understand the logic of propositions, such as "a stitch in time saves nine." They are acquiring new thinking abilities to deal with symbols, so that they can now take courses in algebra, and they are learning how to manipulate many variables at once, allowing them to draw up a budget for their allowance or to plan a study schedule for the week. But all these abilities are new and unfamiliar. They are struggling with their new thinking abilities as much as with their changing bodies. They are often as awkward intellectually as they are physically, and an insensitive remark such as "You're losing your hair, aren't you?" reflects only their intellectual inexperience. How can we ignore this inexperience and not recruit a psychotherapist to think along with them to rescue them from the toxic thinking of depression? Most of them can't go it alone.

But psychotherapy might not easily be obtainable for most adolescents. In a 1999 report on mental health, the U.S. surgeon general said, "Many barriers remain that prevent children, teenagers, and their parents from seeking help from the small number of specially trained professionals."

The era of managed mental health care has encouraged the preferential pharmacological treatment of mental illness. In many health plans, visits to the family doctor for the management of antidepressant medications are often reimbursed more generously than visits to a psychotherapist. This is the result of managed care's goal of shifting patient care from specialist physicians to primary care physicians, who tend to use medications for depression rather than recommend psychotherapy. Some insurance contracts limit the number of sessions or days of treatment or set lifetime "caps" for the treatment of mental illnesses. Another trend in managed care is to subcontract the coverage for mental health care to a "carve-out" insurer. This is a "specialty insurer" that often tries to reduce costs by limiting the number of visits that a depressed patient may make both to a primary care physician and to a psychotherapist.

And millions of Americans have no health insurance whatsoever.

Worse than limited accessibility is the limited numbers of mental health professionals who specialize in adolescent issues. In fact, the statistics are alarming:

- There are currently about 6,700 child and adolescent psychiatrists practicing in this country, although various surveys in the past decade have estimated the current need to be somewhere between 12,000 and 30,000.

- Fewer graduating medical students are choosing training in child and adolescent psychiatry, and the number of training programs is decreasing.
- About one-third of U.S. medical students receive minimal or no training in child and adolescent psychiatry, and so they are incapable of filling the void left by the paucity of child and adolescent psychiatrists.
- Other kinds of mental health professionals who treat depression—psychologists, psychiatric social workers, and marriage and family therapists—are in short supply, too. There simply are not enough mental health professionals to go around.
- There is a serious maldistribution of psychotherapeutic services. Teenagers in rural areas or impoverished areas have significantly reduced access to an adolescent therapist.

Even when mental health care can be accessed, teenagers are notorious for poor compliance with it. They often are too uncomfortable or embarrassed to discuss emotional issues, and they fear a breach of confidentiality that could mean their peers will discover their secret. Their stage of emotional maturation makes some of the psychotherapy discussions seem incomprehensible or useless. They often resent the status of "patient" as a denial of the independence from adults that they are trying to achieve. Perhaps the worst deterrent to a teenager's continuing with psychotherapy is the unfortunate stigma that is attached to depression. Teens are preoccupied with their image and fear they will be perceived as "crazy" or "psycho."

Tragically, the depressed teenagers who are the worst at compliance with mental health care are the most seriously depressed—those who have attempted suicide. These are the statistics for our young people. If you think your teenager is depressed, you might want to sit down. Fifteen percent of adolescents who attempt suicide never keep a single follow-up appointment with a psychotherapist. Only 30 percent keep one or two appointments. In other words, about half of the teenagers who attempt suicide will have at most two fifty-minute conversations with a therapist about the shattered condition of their psyche. Two conversations don't amount to a Band-Aid. Even more distressing are reports that 9 percent of high school students and 10 percent of college freshman have made at least one suicide attempt, and many of them will make a repeat attempt in a year or so.

The message for parents of depressed teenagers couldn't be clearer.

They must forge partnerships. Mental health professionals are in short supply. In an attempt to control costs, some insurance contracts may limit access to them even when they can be found. Also, depressed teenagers are reluctant to keep appointments with them and may drop out of therapy prematurely. Parents must fill the void, and parents are uniquely qualified to do so. Dr. Jerry Rushton, an adolescent-medicine specialist affiliated with the University of Michigan Depression Center, made this plea last year: "We must turn outside the box. Partnering with mental health professionals is the key today to better treatment."

"Most demons—most forms of anguish—rely on the cover of night," wrote Andrew Solomon in the moving chronicle of his own depression, *Noonday Demon*. "To see them clearly is to defeat them." For a child's anguish, can you think of a better candleholder than a parent?

The Best Parent for the Job

Once you recognize the mandate for parental partnering, it's time to make a decision about who will be the primary partner. In some cases both parents can share equally in the responsibility, but far more often one person has to take the lead. It should still be a team effort, but the team needs a captain who oversees the strategic plan. Having one person in charge reduces confusion and conflict. Think of expectant couples who naively plan that they will take equal care of the baby once it arrives. Nine times out of ten, one parent, usually the mother, ends up doing the lion's share of the child care. Arguments and frustration can be avoided if the couple discuss the reality of the situation beforehand and come to a workable agreement about how they will apportion the responsibilities.

Unlike baby care, however, when it comes to partnering for teenage depression, it's not necessarily the mother who is best equipped for the job. Sometimes mothers are too emotionally invested in their child's happiness to deal with the depression dispassionately. Or the mother might be the parent with whom the adolescent has the stormier relationship. Or the mother might be too busy with her career, or with taking care of younger children or elderly parents.

A number of variables and criteria must be considered when making the decision about who will be the main parental partner for the depressed teenager.

Who has fewer conflicts with the teen? Quite often, teenagers will choose the parent with whom they were closer as young children. Obviously, if one parent is now constantly fighting with the teenager, the other is a better candidate.

Who has more compassion? A parent who thinks the teenager should just "pull himself up by the bootstraps" is not going to have the compassion required for the delicate art of partnering.

Who will be the stronger advocate for the teenager? Compassion must be coupled with assertiveness, since the partnering parent may need to advocate for the teenager with school personnel, therapists, and physicians.

Who is more sensitive to the teen's inner life? Often one parent, by virtue of gender, personality traits, intellectual understanding, or intuition, has a better understanding of the teen's inner life.

Who has better rapport with the teen? Often both sensitivity to the teenager's inner life and rapport in day-to-day living are related to which of the four dyads is involved: mother-daughter, mother-son, father-son, or father-daughter. Not surprisingly, the mother-daughter dyad is generally considered to be the closest relationship, followed by father-son, mother-son, then father-daughter. However, during the topsy-turvy teenage years, it's not as simple as deciding that the parent with the "best" dyadic relationship to the teen ought to take charge of the partnering. Sometimes the mother-daughter relationship becomes so fraught with emotional intensity and pain that it is impossible for the mother to set aside her feelings enough to be sufficiently objective about partnering. Or the father-son relationship might become a power struggle, with the son rebelling furiously against his father's well-intentioned efforts. Consider the dynamics in your own family and weigh all the factors before appointing the chief parental partner.

Which parent is not in denial? Sometimes, parents find it virtually impossible to accept that the child they worked so hard to raise and love so much is actually depressed. While understandable, a parent in denial is a poor candidate to be the lead partner. The partnering parent must accept that the teenager is depressed and that depression is an illness, not merely a bad mood, an attitude problem, or a passing phase.

Which parent feels more hopeful about the partnering approach to teenage depression? Partnering is arduous and is best undertaken with conviction. While no one expects you to have blind faith, the parent-partner should be optimistic about this process. Don't try to convince a skeptical spouse by yourself; let him read this book and hear from parents who have successfully rescued their teenagers using these strategies. Then decide which of you is better equipped to lead the effort.

Which parent has the less demanding schedule? Partnering requires the willingness and ability to adapt your schedule according to your teenager's needs. This is one of the biggest hurdles for today's

Parental Partner Checklist

To decide who is better qualified to take on the role of parental partner, you and your spouse should answer the following questions. Yes answers indicate that you have the right attributes. No one is perfect, and you don't have to answer yes to all the questions to qualify. The spouse with the greater number of yes answers will likely be the more successful partner in implementing the strategies against depression.

❏ Do you feel a strong and unconditional love for the teenager, despite any ongoing conflicts?

❏ Do you now—or did you before the depression—have good rapport with the teen?

❏ Do you accept that your teenager is depressed?

❏ Do you feel compassionate toward the teenager, even when dealing with your own anger and frustration?

❏ Do you feel that you can be a strong advocate for your child, if needed?

❏ Do you believe that parental partnering can play a crucial role in recovery from teenage depression?

❏ Does your schedule allow you time to implement the partnering strategies?

❏ Are you willing and able to adjust your schedule as needed?

❏ Do you have daily or near daily access to the teenager?

❏ Are you free of addictions?

❏ Is your own health strong and stable enough to take on this responsibility?

Your score_____ Your spouse's score_____

time-crunched parents. The parent who takes on the job of partnering may have to cut back on work hours or seek more flexibility in the work schedule.

Which parent is free of addictions? An adult who is mired in addiction of any kind, whether it's alcohol, drugs, or behavioral, is not well qualified to be the parental partner. Addictions will rob the adult of the selflessness and focus required for the job. Moreover, the partnering attempts may be rejected by a teenager who is harboring resentment and disappointment over a parent's addiction.

Which parent is in good physical health? A parent suffering from a chronic physical illness needs to assess whether this condition will interfere with acting as the lead partner. A supportive role might be more appropriate for the parent whose energy and activities are curtailed by chronic illness.

Which parent in a divorced family lives with the teenager? In general, the birth parent who lives with the teenager is the better person to be the primary partner, but if the teenager is alienated from that custodial parent, and the noncustodial birth parent lives nearby and has full access, perhaps a successful shared partnering can be negotiated.

Notes for Divorced Parents

Right now, 35 percent of teenagers will become part of a stepfamily before they turn eighteen. And there's little doubt that stepparents treat stepchildren differently from biological children.

Forty years ago, theoretical biologist W. D. Hamilton said that part of the explanation was genetic. With an elegant scientific and mathematical analysis, he showed that altruistic behavior between any two individuals is determined by the degree of genetic relatedness between them. Thus, parents favor their own genetic material, and they will protect their children more than their grandchildren, and grandchildren more than great-grandchildren. Another part of the explanation is psychological. Simply put, we have a natural emotional attachment for biological children over stepchildren. In fact, a recent thought-provoking survey showed that about 15 percent of stepparents fail to mention stepchildren when asked to identify all family members living in the household. In the same survey, 30 percent of stepchildren failed to mention the residential stepparent.

So, if you have a depressed stepchild, you may have to work at overcoming "Hamilton's Rule" and your natural emotional tendencies.

Often, stepfathers withdraw from stepchildren because they feel hurt after their overtures to stepchildren early in the remarriage are rebuffed or ignored. In addition, stepfathers are sometimes hesitant to become close to their stepchildren because they fear that their biological children will feel betrayed. Even though stepfathers are often astute observers of dysfunctional family dynamics, they may allow themselves to become outsiders with little authority and voice. They end up passive, sacrificing what they know is best for their stepchildren. That must change. The children of divorce do best when loved by many adults.

Stepmothers get endowed with a largely undeserved negative cultural stereotype. Still, some studies show that children living with stepmothers are less likely to have routine doctor visits or established places for routine health care, important factors when it comes to medically screening a teenager for depression and detecting it early. This tendency is reversed if stepchildren have regular contact with their birth mothers.

The situation for a parent whose depressed biological child resides in a stepfamily can be especially difficult. When a birth parent is absent from the scene, addressing the problem may require a solution that is not for the immature or selfish, nor for the faint of heart. It is called coparenting.

Coparenting is "divorce family-style," a term popularized by journalist Melinda Blau, who wrote a definitive book about it. Long recognized is that the children of divorce do best when cared for by both birth parents, because parents have immense power, and two parents have twice the power of one. In coparenting, the birth parents establish a cooperative arrangement for dividing parenting time for the child, ignoring living arrangements and allocation of time, if necessary, and working around or even "above" formal custody decrees. The family reorganizes into one that spans two households, the so-called binuclear family, ensuring that one parent will not be forever lost to the child. Communication about major issues in the teen's life, including the course of the depression, is the crucial second aspect of coparenting, and so the parents must set up a regular conference schedule with each other. If ongoing discord prevents this, pickup and drop-off times should provide a good opportunity for face-to-face communication. If divorced parents can't talk at all, letters or e-mail are still useful.

"Impossible" is often the initial reaction to the idea of coparenting. After all, divorced parents need a long time to work out anger, resentment, and hurt, if they ever can. Still, statistics show that fully half of divorced couples are eventually capable of putting in place some kind of substantive arrangement for shared parenting. Time seems to heal the wounds of divorce a bit, and the more time that has elapsed since the divorce decree, the greater is the chance that a coparenting arrangement will be possible.

The crisis of teenage depression should speed the progression toward coparenting. When a child is in trouble, the adults need to set aside their own agendas and do what is best for their teenager. One parent may have to initiate a coparenting arrangement, even in the face of resistance. Fortunately, a persistent and energetic initiative often changes the attitude of the resistant ex-spouse.

Perhaps the most difficult obstacle to coparenting is the alienated or rejecting child. This kind of teenager is not ambivalent at all—she hates and resents the divorced parent. The father is usually the target, and he hears her recite an incessant litany of grievances against him. It's painful and difficult to withstand. Nonetheless, the father should doggedly persist in establishing regular contact with the alienated teen.

Depressed teenagers are exceptionally needy. They feel powerless and crave evidence that people of power have been recruited into their fight. The alienated teenager's acknowledgment of her father's help may not come for years, if ever. But on some level coparenting will assure a depressed teen that both parents are watching, and that she will not fall through the cracks into endless despair.

The Ten Parental Partnering Strategies

Once you've decided who's going to be the chief parental partner, or the lead member of the team, you'll want to begin as soon as possible. It's likely that you've watched your teenager suffer for a long time, you've felt the frustration of standing by helplessly, and you're eager to act. The ten Parental Partnering Strategies for teen depression will give you a framework:

- *Strategy One: See through the disguises of teenage depression.* See behind the masks of teenage depression and learn to differentiate depression from "normal" misbehavior and mood swings.
- *Strategy Two: Add up the clues.* Understand the classic symptoms and the more subtle signs of depression.
- *Strategy Three: Identify related problems—depression's companions.* Look for symptoms of comorbid conditions such as anxiety, anorexia,

ADHD, oppositional-defiant disorder, OCD, substance abuse, bipolar disorder, and dysthymia.

- *Strategy Four: Be alert to suicide risk and practice suicide prevention.* Learn to detect signs of suicidal tendencies, cope with suicide gestures, and prevent suicide attempts.

- *Strategy Five: Work with your family physician and manage the medications.* Monitor the side effects and track the benefits of antidepressants and other medications.

- *Strategy Six: Find the right therapist.* Identify the best physician and therapist, and navigate the medical system and health insurance labyrinth.

- *Strategy Seven: Take the family inventory.* Assess if and how the family is contributing to the depression, and work on unresolved family issues.

- *Strategy Eight: Bring the "talking cure" home.* Break through adolescent anger and resentment to establish good communication and serve as your teenager's "therapist at home."

- *Strategy Nine: Look beyond therapy.* Consider adjunctive practices such as exercise, meditation, and yoga, as well as the importance of diet, sleep, and spirituality.

- *Strategy Ten: Consider schools and schedules.* Choose a nurturing school and guide your teenager through the transition to college life.

While the Parental Partnering Strategies are not quick fixes or miracle cures, they have proven to elicit substantial results. Parents and clinicians across a wide spectrum have found that these techniques work. The following ten chapters will give you the tools you need to implement these strategies to lead your teenager out of depression.

Part 2

The Ten Strategies of Parental Partnering

3

Strategy One
See through the Disguises of Teenage Depression

Teenage depression is often a wily impostor. Adolescents are confusing at best, and even more so when they are depressed. At least half the time teenage depression masks itself. That's why turning yourself into an ace detective is the first strategy of parental partnering.

The typical depressed adult seems to have stepped back from life, exhibiting flattened emotions, sad or blank facial expressions, intellectual slowness, lack of enthusiasm, and energy that is hard to muster and easily dissipated. These are the signs we ordinarily expect to see with depression, and when present, there is usually no mistaking the malicious fog that has enveloped the person. But depressed teenagers often look much different. Don't necessarily expect to see them sighing and moping all the time, and succumbing to frequent fits of crying.

Teenage depression often wears a disguise, but the disguise can be undone with the powers of careful observation. Take a lesson from Arthur Conan Doyle, who endowed Sherlock Holmes with these talents. Actually, Conan Doyle used one of his own Edinburgh medical school professors, Dr. Joseph Bell, as the model for Holmes's razor-sharp deductive capacities. "Use your eyes, sir! Use your ears, use your brain, and your bump of perception," Dr. Bell would exhort his students. Dr. Bell was famous among his medical colleagues for his ability to discern habits, occupations, and diseases—even diagnose afflictions without ever laying his hands upon the patient. Like Dr. Bell, you must recruit your powers of observation. And they are indeed *powers,* because only parents are so carefully tuned in to their teenager's behavior.

Don't Rely on Others to Do Your Detective Work

No one else can be as good a detective as a parent. No matter how tempted you might be, don't rely on anyone else. Period.

For years now, the medical profession itself has admitted that primary care doctors are poor screeners for depression, and simply because they often omit the screen from their routine examination. In fact, the latest statistics show that at least 60 percent of teenage depression is never diagnosed. The situation is so critical that a task force sponsored by the Department of Health and Human Services exhorted primary care doctors to screen formally for depression. Unfortunately, this screen comprises only two questions: "Over the past two weeks have you ever felt down, depressed, or helpless?" And, "Have you felt little interest or pleasure in doing things?" Although the task force's effort is commendable, it's woefully insufficient.

To make matters worse, "doctors don't want to hear about

depression," says John Greden, executive director of the Depression Center at the University of Michigan Medical School. Although counterproductive, some of their motives, he says, spring from true patient concern. One is to avoid stigmatizing the patient with the label *depressed*. Instead, the doctor may conclude that the patient is "stressed," "exhausted," or perhaps has "low blood sugar." Another motive is to preserve future insurability for mental health care.

Many physicians still get caught in the trap of assuming that depression is not an illness but merely a "state of mind." A National Mental Health Association survey last year revealed that one-third of doctors cling to this antiquated idea. The bottom line—you can't rely on your family doctor to do the initial screening.

Teachers and school counselors can't be counted on to be first to recognize teen depression, either. Many adolescents put on a convincing show at school so as not to appear sad and needy in front of their peers, and the depression may only manifest once the curtain is down and they go home. In addition, teachers and even counselors are often ill-equipped to ferret out the disguises or subtleties of teen depression. One student, Chloe, described how school personnel dismissed her depression at the beginning of the tenth grade, not once but twice. "I started crying spontaneously in history class, but I didn't know why. The history teacher asked me to stay around after the class—but asked me if I had a problem using drugs." To make matters worse, when Chloe's depression was finally diagnosed, her counselor at school fell prey to the myth of depression being incongruous with youth and beauty. "The counselor said I'm a bright and attractive young lady. She told me, 'You've got all these good things going for you. You're fine. You're young.'"

Your teenager's friends, even a best friend, won't usually clue you in either. Teenagers try to avoid talking to adults about uncomfortable topics such as emotional health. And since they have the same immature thinking capacities as your son or daughter, they will have just as hard a time recognizing depression in others as in themselves.

Clearly, you can't depend on your teenager's physician, teachers, counselors, or friends to do the detective work. It's up to you to put together the clues and then take the initiative to bring your child to a health-care professional for further evaluation. But before you're ready to employ your deductive powers, you have to take stock of your own attitudes and make sure that they've created no blind spots.

Beware the Blinders: Reluctance, Guilt, Denial, and Fear

Are you reluctant to say out loud to your spouse that you think your teenager might be depressed? Are you afraid even to allow the idea entry into your own private thoughts? Are you reluctant to ask your teenager the necessary probing questions to find out if he or she is depressed?

Most of the parents whom I interviewed for this book were reluctant. I was, too. Guilt is the biggest reason—and it's universal among parents of depressed teenagers. Lauren's mother is convinced she is a huge cause of her daughter's depression. "I'm guilty about the parenting I did when she was little," she said. "I think I taught her how to be sad. I spent a lot of my life feeling odd, feeling like the odd man out. When I got messages that Lauren felt that way, I felt like a failure."

Other parents feel guilty because they think they might have contributed "faulty" genes to their child. Chloe knows her father feels this way because of the mental illness within their family. "My father is a manic-depressive," she said. "The family tried to keep it a secret. Sometimes he would pretend to speak in Spanish even though he knew no Spanish. We couldn't keep it a secret then. And my brother is a schizophrenic." In fact, data from adoption studies consistently show higher rates of depression among adopted children whose birth parents had experienced depression. Yes, there is a genetic factor.

Perhaps you're reluctant because you are a stepparent. Toss that excuse out right away. Stepparents are often the most astute observers of family relationships and family dynamics. You have every right to make observations and take steps to safeguard the mental health of a stepchild.

You may be reluctant because you know that facing up to your child's depression will cause *you* sadness. This was my case with Eric. I knew there was going to be no instant rescue. And I knew that for him the depression would be a series of detours, some of them long and exasperating for both of us. While other teens were thinking about careers or colleges, Eric would be struggling to find a reason to get out of bed. While other teens were planning on asking dates to proms or to football games, Eric was trying to get up the nerve to talk to a salesclerk. And while others were preparing for the SAT or the ACT, Eric was desperately trying to stay awake in class after another insomniac night.

Maybe you are denying the depression because you can't accept that perhaps your parenting skills failed to produce a happy, well-adjusted teen.

I understand that one, too. I was assiduous, maybe even compulsive, in stockpiling and practicing good parenting skills. My wife, Patricia, was equally conscientious and loving, if not more so. How the hell could this then be happening to Eric? And to us? Impossible! Then, too, I was afraid of the social stigma, convinced that other parents would look at us accusingly. After all, parents are taught early on to take a large measure of credit for their children's successes, and an even larger measure for their failures. Depression could be looked upon as a failure, even though I knew better. That's when my sadness turned to anger. I felt cheated.

Lauren's mother felt cheated, too. "How could I have put this much effort into it and not have it come out the way I wanted it to?" she said. Worse, you may even worry that your teen's depression might indicate parental malfeasance.

Now here's the hardest one to swallow. Maybe you're denying it because you know, deep down, that family dysfunctions can contribute to teenage depression. Well, get ready. Breathe slowly, or turn on a fan. You're right. Parental addictions, marital conflicts, teen-parent conflicts, physical or verbal abuse, and many other unfortunate dysfunctions promote or perpetuate teen depression. That's why taking a family inventory is one of the Ten Strategies of Parental Partnering.

The adage is right: "Feel the fear and do it anyway." Don't delay. You have to begin your detective work *now*. The science is in: early diagnosis and early treatment make a huge difference in the long-term outlook for teen depression. The sooner an episode of major depression is diagnosed and treated, the less is the likelihood of a recurrence of major depression. Moreover, delayed treatment may allow the depression to convert to an especially nasty form that can recur even in the absence of a trigger.

If you think your teenager is depressed, you've got an urgent situation on your hands. You have to be the adult and set aside your denial, guilt, and fear. Get busy with your detective work and read on to learn how to recognize the many masks of teen depression.

The Mask of Anger

The most frequent disguise of teen depression is intensely off-putting for parents. It is an angry or irritable mood, often coupled with rebellious behavior. Teens normally get irritable at times because of the dramatic changes that are occurring in their bodies, their thinking capacities, and their station in life. An irritability that becomes pervasive or is repeatedly out of proportion to the provocation is definitely abnormal. Many of these chronically irritable teenagers, doctors say, are actually depressed, and the degree of irritability often indicates the degree of depression.

The irritability seems to be a substitute for depression's sadness, yet the reasons for this are unclear. Some adolescent psychologists say that depression is a discomfort teenagers cannot identify. It is so confusing to teenagers' limited abilities for abstract thought that they react with anger and hostility simply because they don't know what else to do.

In some cases, the irritability mutates into anger, and the angry outbursts may even be explosive and dangerous. "Matthew was wild, uncontrollable, and hostile," his father said. "Everything bothered him. One night my wife and I were in bed asleep. Matthew jumped on me and started choking me. He was five eleven and weighed about two hundred and fifteen [pounds]. We called the police and had him arrested. It was one of the hardest things I had to do, especially since I was his stepfather. Later I found out we could have had an intervention where the police come to the house to calm him down and say they will take him away if it happens again. But that time, he stayed in jail overnight."

Irritability and anger may surface as rebellious behavior such as truancy, staying out past curfews, or running away from home. In teenage boys, these emotions may manifest as antisocial behavior such as bullying, getting into fights, vandalism, theft, or forcing someone into sexual activity. The most worrisome of all is the risk-taking behavior, since teens may not fully comprehend the dangerous or deadly consequences of unprotected sex or illicit drug use.

Many depressed girls, in contrast, direct the anger and hostility inward. They become unresponsive, sullen, and silent. Their very silence can be the loudest cry for help. Alternatively, some depressed teenage girls become extremely "fresh" and verbally hostile with their parents, saying intentionally hurtful things to express their rage. It can be devastating to parents when their daughters who were once such precious little girls become surly to the point of verbal abuse. These parents are often heard to say, "Make her ten again."

The Chameleon Syndrome

A quirk of teenage depression that seriously challenges a parent's detective powers—and patience—is what I call the "chameleon syndrome": a depressed teenager's mood may suddenly change colors depending on the circumstances.

My son Eric was angry and obstreperous at home, picking fights with his mother incessantly, often about inconsequential matters. "We fought every morning in the car while I drove him to school," his mother said. "He complained that I was trashing my car because I ate breakfast in it and maybe dropped a few crumbs. He complained that the floor mats were dirty, and it was that relentless kind of complaining where he wouldn't back off. If I asked him how he was doing in school or whether he was making friends, he would yell and ask why I was prying. It was a horrible two years. It took only a twenty-minute drive each morning to get me near tears and make me feel we were never going to be close again."

At the same time, insatiably argumentative Eric was a model teenager at school. He even won an award his first year in high school for being the most congenial and warmhearted student there. He performed well for adults other than his mother and father.

"Other parents would tell me what a delightful child I had," his mother said. "They said they wished they had one just like him." They never saw the side that his mother and I did.

While Eric was busy hiding his homebound anger with exemplary behavior elsewhere, Lauren's chameleon syndrome forced her to hide her sadness and sense of worthlessness under layers of attractive cosmetics and clothing. Lauren is a comely young lady, an honor student, and an accomplished cross-country athlete, but somehow she had convinced herself she was worthless. "She would refute compliments I gave her," Lauren's mother said. "She would say, 'No, no, I'm not nice. I can't do anything right. I feel like I'm rotten inside.' I asked her once what she saw when she looked in the mirror. She said, 'I see an ugly girl.' I asked her what about that girl was ugly. 'Everything,' she said. Lauren was feeling so bad about herself on the inside that she tried to look better on the outside, and it took me quite a while to figure this out. She used lots of makeup and made sure her makeup was perfect. She would cry on the way to school if she forgot her mascara. She subscribed to three or four fashion magazines. She would plan out a whole week of what she was going to wear, and she kept the plan in a notebook with a grid for each day. Everything was on the grid—clothes, shoes, makeup, hair."

To distract herself and others from how terrible she felt inside, fifteen-year-old Chloe became a chameleon, too, and donned a Greenwich Village kind of disguise. "I made myself look so hip," she said. "I wore poet shirts or broom skirts with elaborate patterns or mirrors glued on them. I wore big vests and put a lot of energy into my jewelry. My favorite was a necklace with bells that made noise when I moved. I used all that as a disguise to look better than I felt. My teachers didn't think I was depressed. They thought I was 'interesting' and avant-garde."

Dangerous Distracters

Depressed teenagers sometimes develop psychosomatic problems. Instead of complaining about sadness, they complain of a headache, abdominal pain, or fatigue. The parent promptly takes the teenager to the family doctor, who conducts an extensive and expensive workup. Often, no cause for the problem is found, and the whole thing is dismissed as nothing more than a transitory condition or something connected to "growing up." Sadly, depression may never get mentioned, let alone diagnosed.

Another common distracter is alcohol or drug abuse, and about 20 percent of depressed teenagers first come to their parents' or doctor's attention this way. The substance abuse is usually an attempt at self-medication to counteract depression's intensely uncomfortable feelings. Parents may focus on the substance abuse as the primary problem when, in fact, it is the consequence of undiagnosed depression.

The distracter of sexual promiscuity causes parents the most consternation. Both depressed girls and boys might engage in promiscuous sex to achieve intimacy when they feel isolated or to achieve self-esteem when they feel worthless. As with substance abuse, focusing on the increased sexual activity as the problem misses the point, since it is primarily a consequence of the core problem of depression.

Is Your Teenager Disguising a Depression?

Instructions: Circle yes or no for each question.

1. Does your teenager seem overly angry?   Yes   No

2. Does your teenager seem overly irritable?   Yes   No

3. Is your teenager overly rebellious?   Yes   No

4. Does your teenager act aggressively?   Yes   No

5. Does your teenager abuse drugs or alcohol?   Yes   No

6. Is your teenager sexually promiscuous?   Yes   No

7. Does your teenager act sullen and silent?   Yes   No

8. Does your teenager say disrespectful or
   cruel things to you?   Yes   No

9. Does your teenager behave well at school
   but poorly at home?   Yes   No

10. Is your teenager overly worried
    about his or her appearance?   Yes   No

11. Does your teenager have frequent headaches,
    vague stomachaches, or fatigue?   Yes   No

Scoring

Count one point for each yes answer circled, then add up the total.

Interpreting the Score

1 point—The item you circled could be only a bad habit, but admittedly an obnoxious or potentially dangerous one. Still, you must keep the possibility of depression in mind, and take this assessment again next month to see if the score worsens.

2 points—It's time to worry and look closer. Depression is a real possibility here. Make sure you take the two assessments in the next chapter on the symptoms and triggers of depression.

3 points or more—It's time to make an appointment for your teen with your family doctor for a formal depression evaluation.

The Myths of Adolescence

A number of myths about adolescence make it more difficult to see through the disguises of teenage depression. The most destructive of these fictions is the myth of teen turmoil. The idea that the adolescent years are a time of "normal" turmoil has done incredible damage to the emotional health of our children, since it is a huge cause of delayed or missed diagnoses. As a parent who is skilled in the art of detection, you need to be aware of how this myth emerged and how it distorts reality.

Several decades ago, well-meaning psychologists unintentionally invented the myth of teen turmoil by studying troubled young people—but generalizing their conclusions to *all* adolescents. They studied a specific group of young people who had mental health problems or conduct disorders, then extrapolated these findings to all teenagers! It's no wonder the findings indicated that teen turmoil was universal. Normal tendencies, these researchers said, could include intense rebellion against authority or the abandonment of sound family values to embrace the idiosyncratic ones of a dysfunctional peer group. Moreover, mood aberrations were alleged to be typical and not necessarily a cause for alarm. The normal adolescent was painted as a fearsome and tempest-tossed creature: hostile, frightened, unpredictable, and moody. Thus, many parents came to believe that happiness was not the normal state of teenagers.

However, well-designed new studies show that the majority of teenagers—about 85 percent—make a smooth transition to adulthood without significant conflicts or turmoil. This doesn't mean that they don't have their periods of moodiness and irritability, nor that the majority of teenagers are perfect saints who never annoy their parents with back talk or rebellion against rules. It does mean that a *persistently* depressed or irritable mood just isn't normal.

This myth of adolescent turmoil is especially pernicious because it gets compounded with a couple of misconceptions. One is that a teenager "outgrows" problems. Maybe yes, but maybe no. If your teenager's mood or behavior is worrisome, you need to translate your worry into action—such as medical attention. That persistent "funky" behavior may not be a quirk or two, but rather a sign of a depressive illness that won't be outgrown. Another misconception is the inevitability of the generation gap. I don't believe for a minute that parents and teenagers are plugged into an unavoidable destiny to misunderstand each other. I do believe, though, that they don't communicate enough. Our schedules, parents' and teens' alike, are stuffed with commitments. There's little time to talk. And when we do, often we don't take our teenager's problems seriously. This is the number one complaint teenagers have about their parents, according to many experts.

A second myth is that a depressed teenager will be able to tell you if he or she is depressed. That's seldom the case, because, by definition, teens are not sophisticated thinkers and have difficulty putting abstract problems such as depression into words. Most teenagers do not yet have the concepts or the vocabulary to accurately describe to parents the painful mystery inside them. Michelle would say, "Something is wrong, but I can't explain it." Blake would say, "I know I'm different, but I don't know why I'm different." "Jared never said anything about his emotions," his mother said. "It wasn't until he was twenty-two that he first used the word *depressed*."

Teenagers also have a knack for misattributing responsibility. They often don't comprehend the internal source of the discomfort and so try to pin it on an external cause. Parents, teachers, and siblings become favorite scapegoats. Adolescents convince themselves that the source of the mysterious and unidentified distress may be their teachers ("They're picking on me") or their peers ("They all think they're better than I am") rather than a terrible glitch in their emotional health. In fact, a sixteen-year-old and only slightly overweight Michelle concluded, according to her father, "The world doesn't like me because I'm fat. I want liposuction." Actually, Michelle was disliked because her behavior was atrocious and her mood disorder made others around her uncomfortable. But Michelle never said she was depressed simply because she couldn't yet understand that. It's fortunate her parents didn't wait for her pronouncement.

The third myth that must be discarded is the notion that depression is a midlife or old-age illness, brought on by the stresses of marriage and career or by the hovering prospect of senescence. It is quite the contrary. Young people actually have an inordinate vulnerability to depression. Doctors who have studied depression in people under the age of forty have determined that the risk of depression is *inversely* related to age. In other words, the people at the greatest risk for this dark and debilitating illness are the youngest. They are our children. In fact, depression is so common among high-school-age students that in a hypothetical high school in the United States today, with an enrollment of a thousand teenagers, *seventy-four cases* of depression could be diagnosed during any given school year.

It's no wonder that teachers, counselors, and community resources are overwhelmed and often miss the crucial signs of teenage depression. Only a parent can be expected to have the insight and determination required to put together the clues and get prompt medical help for a teenager who may otherwise go undiagnosed and untreated. A teen who is struggling is a teen who needs help.

4

Strategy Two
Add Up the Clues

Now comes another challenge for a partnering parent—and it's a tough one. You've got to put all the clues together. Fortunately, the American Psychiatric Association has formulated a definitive checklist that will help you figure out whether your suspicion is well-founded. To qualify as a major depressive episode, the Association says, your teen must show at least one of the two core symptoms: anhedonia, or a depressed or irritable mood.

Anhedonia manifests itself as a significant lack of interest in most or all activities of the day, and an inability to derive pleasure from them. This symptom often quickly evolves into boredom, apathy, or lack of attention.

Only about half of depressed teens will plainly demonstrate a sad mood. "When Lauren was in the ninth grade, she was always crying," her mother said. "She would cry at the littlest things, and her crying was uncontrollable. She would overreact to things that were no big deal, like unloading the dishwasher. I had put her down as being just an extremely sensitive girl." Unfortunately, Lauren's mother didn't try to figure out her crying, but the explanation soon came clear when Lauren made a suicide gesture by jumping off a second-story deck.

The other half of depressed teens don't seem sad at all, and instead they are irritable or angry. Michelle showed both core symptoms. One night, in the midst of a rebellious and defiant outburst, she couldn't stop sobbing and needed to be hospitalized.

The American Psychiatric Association's checklist includes seven additional symptoms, and a truly depressed teenager will show at least four of them:

- A weight loss or a weight gain, or an increase or decrease in appetite
- Difficulty falling asleep at night or difficulty awakening in the morning
- Slowed movements and thinking or, conversely, agitated movements and thinking
- Fatigue or loss of energy
- Feelings of worthlessness or excessive guilt
- Diminished ability to think or concentrate
- Recurrent thoughts of death, recurrent thoughts of suicide, formulation of a suicide plan, or an actual suicide attempt

Now you might be saying to yourself, "I had some of those very things yesterday, and I don't think I'm depressed. What good is this checklist?" That's the point. You must go beyond the checklist. First, the core symptoms and the additional symptoms must be present every day, or nearly every day, for at least two weeks. Second, and more importantly, the symptoms must significantly impair your child's functioning. In other words, depressed teenagers will be struggling or failing at their "jobs." These jobs are performing at school and fitting into their family and peer groups. Poor school grades, a change in grades, chronic absenteeism, withdrawal from family or friends, or isolation are manifestations that shout to a parent that the teenager is depressed.

Here's another caveat. Some depressive episodes are not primary illnesses at all, but rather secondary ones caused directly by a phys-

Does Your Teenager Have the Symptoms of Major Depression?

Instructions: Circle yes or no for each item.

Core Symptoms

1. Depressed or irritable mood for most of the day, nearly every day   Yes   No
2. Markedly diminished interest or pleasure in most activities   Yes   No

Additional Symptoms

3. Significant weight loss, weight gain, decrease or increase in appetite   Yes   No
4. Insomnia (difficulty sleeping) or hypersomnia (sleeping too much)   Yes   No
5. Agitation or, conversely, slowed movements   Yes   No
6. Fatigue or loss of energy   Yes   No
7. Feelings of worthlessness or inappropriate guilt   Yes   No
8. Diminished ability to think, concentrate, and make decisions   Yes   No
9. Recurrent thoughts of death or suicide   Yes   No

Scoring

If you circled yes for at least one of the two core symptoms and yes for at least four of the additional symptoms, your teenager meets the official criteria for depression. An urgent visit to the family doctor is necessary, because your teenager is in significant emotional pain.

If you circled yes for item 9, make an emergency appointment with your family doctor. Your teenager is at risk right now for attempting suicide.

ical illness or substance abuse. Matthew's depression and his frighteningly aggressive outbursts turned out to be the result of a thyroid disease. "His doctors missed his thyroid problem for three years," his father said. "Once he was started on the right thyroid medicines, his mood and his behavior turned around." That's why, before rushing to a therapist, your teen needs to visit the family physician to make sure there's not an inciting medical problem such as thyroid disease, sleep apnea, migraine headaches, rheumatoid arthritis, or diabetes, just to name a few.

It's also important to understand the role of substance abuse. Doctors estimate that as much as 20 percent of teenage depression is a secondary phenomenon due to substance abuse, especially with tranquilizers, anabolic steroids, painkillers, cocaine, hallucinogens, and, of course, alcohol. If you haven't done it yet, you had better broach this issue now. Alcohol abuse among teenagers is burgeoning, and it's making headlines.

Subtle Symptoms

Sherlock Holmes's role model, Dr. Bell, taught his Edinburgh medical students that "recognition depends in great measure on the accurate and rapid appreciation of the small points." For successful partnering, you, too, must be acutely alert to the small points and the subtle signs. The list of "classic" symptoms above is a good start, but the signs of teenage depression can be subtle and require closer examination to detect.

Anhedonia is one of the two core symptoms of depression, but a teenager may show only minor signs of this symptom. As mentioned, anhedonia is the demoralizing experience that activities that used to produce pleasure no longer do so. Sports, hobbies, music,

TV, family outings, reading, movies, all become bland or stale, and the world seems drained of color. Depressed teens fail to anticipate moments of pleasure, even little ones like driving a first car with the radio on or browsing in a store for clothes. They lose the capacity to imagine the future with anticipation, or to participate in the present with joy.

Unable to find the correct words or concepts to express this peculiar distress, a depressed teenager may complain that activities are "boring" or friends are "dumb." These trifling comments mask a huge distress. Anhedonia steals in and quietly claims the young person who once told the funniest stories, who couldn't wait for basketball season to begin, or who used to adore her dance classes.

Some depressed teens withdraw from friends or extracurricular activities, offering thin or flimsy excuses such as "I don't have time" or "I don't feel well." Even if it doesn't seem like much to go on, trust your intuition. Depressed teens think poorly of themselves, and an insidious cycle may start when they act poorly as a result, with others then judging them adversely on their awkward or seemingly antisocial behavior. The cycle is self-reinforcing and may spiral downward, beyond withdrawal and into social isolation. It's urgent for parents to pick up on the withdrawal before it gets to this stage.

Depressed people are supposed to be slow movers. Some teenagers do look sluggish, but others become fidgety and nervous. Some pace. Some wring their hands. Some nervously wind their hair around their fingers. Eric did all of these, and he chewed his fingernails incessantly, too. Some can't seem to stay still long enough to finish dinner, do a short homework assignment, or even sit through a blockbuster movie. One of the reasons for this is that about half of depressed teenagers are also afflicted with some kind of anxiety syndrome, an accomplice that heaps on a second kind of distress.

It's no wonder that school performance suffers. An inability to pay attention in class and to concentrate on homework drops a grade point average as quickly and as certainly as a month's worth of truancy.

Switching peer groups is a subtle sign parents need especially to heed, because the switch doesn't necessarily mean a change in your teen's values. Rather, the switch is often a compensatory mechanism to evade the pain of the depression. Michelle felt unattractive and sought popularity among those in her school whom she viewed as being less choosy. "Michelle used to be conscientious," her father said. "But she just gave up on it all. She developed an apathy towards school and started hanging out with kids who had no interest in doing well in school."

Eric, too, was short on self-esteem. Although not gay, he started hanging out almost exclusively with the gay and lesbian students at his high school because, as he insisted, they were more tolerant and quicker to accept him since they were having their own kinds of troubles with peer acceptance. Their ready acceptance gave him a measure of comfort in his insecurity, although it ultimately showed itself as nothing more than an illusion of comfort.

A depressed teen's use of an "antidote" for the depression might be the hardest for a parent to figure out. Eric's antidote was caffeine. Although he was already fidgety, he drank huge cups of coffee every morning on the way to school. He was exceptionally sensitive to caffeine, and it made him overly animated and talkative. I nagged him about the coffee-drinking because it made him look nervous, but he said he needed it to look "alive" in front of his friends. Eric used a second antidote, a favorite of many depressed teens: he immersed himself in social activities. The social whirl was a drug of sorts that gave him a dose of temporary amnesia, enabling him to forget the pain and isolation he was feeling. Sadly, all this frenetic activity never enhanced his self-esteem.

Loss of appetite is often associated with adult depression, but the situation for depressed teens may be entirely the opposite. Understandably, teenage obesity seems to promote depression, since body image is so important to teens. But newer studies conducted at the University of Cincinnati Medical Center show the converse is also true—that depression is a major cause of teenage obesity. The doctors who performed the study speculate that treating the depression in this circumstance could reverse the obesity.

Perhaps the most subtle sign is the failure of speech. It can become slow and halting, or monotonous, with long pauses before answers or with perfunctory or repetitious comments peppered into the talk. This is sometimes misinterpreted as teenage apathy. But Kate Millet, who authored an eloquent account of her own depression, says this about the deadening of language: "It is as if the inner voice is so urgent in its discourse—how shall I live?—that there is nothing important to advance by way of conversation." But language does not really go away, she says. It goes inward and downward, shriveling. The depressed teenager mourns the loss of language because she needs sociability and camaraderie now more than ever. In the face of this misery, she does not even have the use of words to protect herself and feels as if she is growing mute as well as hopeless. William Styron wrote that not only could he not think of words, he could not get them out: "I sensed myself turning walleyed, monosyllabic. The ferocious inwardness of the pain produced an immense distraction that prevented my articulating words beyond a hoarse murmur."

Detecting the Pain of Depression

One of the essential tasks for parents who are partners is to be able to recognize and respect the immense pain of depression. When someone has a visible physical illness, injury, or handicap, it's easy to sympathize, but the invisible, yet immeasurable pain of depression is hard to detect and accept.

"Imagine the worst physical pain you've ever had—a broken bone, a toothache, or labor pain," says Dr. Andrew Slaby, an expert on teenage suicide. "Multiply it tenfold and take away the cause. Then you can possibly approximate the mental pain of depression. It can be far more overwhelming, more incapacitating, than any physical pain."

Depression is unimaginable if you've never been depressed yourself. For two of the depressed teenagers in this book, only their creative outlets could begin to describe the terrible feelings.

Blake was sure he had photographed his own depression. He thought he had finally captured the mysterious beast on film and that the picture might explain the torment to his parents or some of his tenth-grade classmates. The day Blake took the picture was frigid and dreary, typical of late winter in Minnesota. He was fulfilling a homework assignment given by his photography teacher to do a self-portrait. Camera in hand, Blake had trekked outside into the cold and paused in front of a barren young tree that seemed fragile against the gusting wind. This could be my stand-in, he thought, but it lacked a crucial detail. So Blake took off his glasses and hung them in the tree, but backward, as if the Blake-tree were being forced to look through the lenses the wrong way. Depression distorts everything I see, his photograph said, and the backwardness of the lenses also distorts what my friends see of me when they look into my eyes.

Lauren was severely depressed in high school, too, and over the course of her depression she would make three suicide gestures, mercifully unsuccessful. Lauren tried to describe its pain in her poetry:

> *Every day, I am brought to the gates of hell.*
> *Every day, I enter the dancing flames.*

I open this salted wound by opening my eyes,
I enter this violence by awakening.
It leaves scars that are too deep for anyone else to see.
It is happening more and more often.

Because ordinary words and images fail to depict their anguish, depressed people often resort to metaphors. Darkness is the most common one—typically a slow but inexorable slide into blindness. Styron calls it a storm of murk. Another much used metaphor is that of falling: a pit or crack on the surface of the earth has suddenly opened up and swallowed the depressed person. The silent, breezeless fall down the abyss is perpetual. Author Rosemary Dinnage likens depression to the insatiable worm inside the bud, gnawing until the "me" is gone to nothingness. Still, Styron insists, all images are off the mark, and not even the best artists can find the right words.

The Twin Demons: Worthlessness and Hopelessness

Depression is not an extreme form of sadness, although sadness is a big part of it. Depression is not grief, because grief has an object such as a lost relationship that is grieved over. Nor is it just a bad case of the "blues" or a huge "funk." Rather, the essence of depression is the sufferer's conviction that he has no value. The abyss down which your teenager might be falling is the unremitting sense of his or her worthlessness.

This sense of worthlessness, accompanied by hopelessness, makes depression genuine anguish. A morbid pessimism makes even small obstacles appear insurmountable. Depressed teenagers perceive their skills as inadequate for the tasks at hand, and this is in great part true. They are not yet mature enough to develop long lists of problem-solving strategies and sensible options for handling the trouble. Consequently, teenagers' efforts at defense or counterattack are often limited and ineffective. Teenage depression is thus especially hurtful owing to the precarious stage of life at which it attacks. In the intensity of adolescence, problems appear so daunting that teenagers are convinced no one possesses sufficient power to rescue them.

Philosophers call depression a disease of the soul because it poisons a person's abilities to reason. A depressed teenager seems dim-witted even to herself. She comes to believe that objects and situations are as unimportant and meaningless as she thinks she herself is. Homework, grooming, piano lessons—why bother? What is the point of getting up in the morning? As a result, any driving sense of purpose withers, and vitality disappears. Too sapped to hunker down, she cowers down into a self-protective mode. Anticipation becomes a joyless thing, because her anticipation is only of pain in the future. Perhaps the cruelest of depression's other dimensions is the choking off of her capacity to give or receive affection: I am so unattractive a person, who could ever want to be my friend? What do my parents really think of me? Why would anyone want to accept the love of a worthless person like me?

Twelve Depression Triggers

Parents can help detect teen depression by looking for triggers. Many diseases have triggers that set off the illness initially or precipitate recurrent attacks. Just ask any parent who has a child with asthma. Psychologically stressful events can suddenly strangle an asthmatic child's breathing so badly that the attack may even turn fatal. The same kind of triggering phenomenon is true for teens with diabetes: stressful triggers may result in poor blood-sugar control.

In hemophiliacs, high emotional arousal can increase the tendency to bleed.

Depression is a disease with its own particular triggers, and parents must be alert to them.

TRIGGER #1: ENTERING A NEW SCHOOL. A graph of the incidence of childhood and teenage depression shows two tall peaks. One occurs when children are just about to enter puberty. The other peak is during the ages of thirteen to fifteen. It is no coincidence that these peaks correspond with the child starting middle school or high school. I'm sure you remember how stressful it was to go to a new school. It is even more so today, since schools have become less nurturing places to form an identity while making the necessarily slow and deliberate transition to adulthood.

TRIGGER #2: FIRST YEAR OF COLLEGE. You've heard at least one of your friends say about their child, "She's just having a bad freshman year." That bad year may actually be a year of paralysis by depression. In fact, U.S. drug companies estimate that during the next five years as many as 1.6 million incoming college freshman will experience an episode of depression. College health officials say that as many as 20 percent of college students will take antidepressant medications during their college years. College freshman have many stresses—academic pressure, romantic woes, too much junk food, too little sleep, difficulties with time management, and independence from parents for the first time. The *New York Times* reported recently that stress on college campuses has increased so much that counseling centers get boomingly busy just two weeks into the academic year.

TRIGGER #3: TOO MUCH HOMEWORK AND ACADEMIC PRESSURE. Homework is the newest of the stressors, because the homework load nowadays is often off the charts. *Wall Street Journal* writer Sue Shellenbarger reported that one seventh-grader in New York wrestled with up to six hours of homework each night. Shellenbarger says the evidence proves that the homework boom is causing student burnout, and she lists these danger signs: chronic irritability, emotional detachment, isolation, or crowded-out hobbies. This kind of burnout may also trigger depression.

TRIGGER #4: TOO MUCH SCHEDULED ACTIVITY. Teens with over-committed schedules burn out, too. Yes, extracurricular activities foster initiative, participation in voluntary sports is associated with better school performance, and a part-time job teaches a teen time management. But if the teen's portfolio is crammed full, the first casualties are family time and family relationships. The largest teen study ever conducted, the National Longitudinal Study of Adolescent Health, involved ninety thousand young people and found that family closeness is linked to less smoking, less alcohol and drug use, and less early sex. Although depression was not specifically identified in this study, it's a good bet that family closeness is also a major player in this realm. It's not just the burnout caused by an overburdened schedule that predisposes to depression, but the concurrent meagerness of family involvement.

TRIGGER #5: INADEQUATE SOCIAL SKILLS OR UNPOPULARITY. Relationships are so important during the teen years that some doctors implicate the inability to get positive reinforcement from peers as sufficient to initiate or maintain a depressed state. This seemed to be part of the explanation for Eric's depression. His social self-confidence was rock-bottom, and he ranked himself as unworthy. He became passive, submissive, hesitant, and pessimistic, but only with his peers. He was robust and confident with adults (other than his parents)—even charming I was told—but relationships with adults count for little with a teen. Eric measured his self-worth by his peer acceptance.

TRIGGER #6: UNATTRACTIVENESS AND SOCIAL REJECTION. Some teenagers are, sadly, unattractive to their peers. They are the loners, the geeks, and the rejects. "Jared has severe ADHD, and he stood out because of his extreme impulsiveness," his mother said. "Kids picked on him constantly. He was rejected from friendships. He was rejected by cousins in our family. He was even rejected by church groups, and I have a real hard time with that one. He doesn't feel valuable because he's been so hurt. Jared has been rejected so many times, there's no place for him to step out."

TRIGGER #7: ACCUMULATION OF SMALL STRESSORS. Little things mean a lot. Child psychologists Barbara Ingersoll and Sam Goldstein wisely note, "Sometimes it isn't one major stressful event that overwhelms a young person's ability to cope and results in a depressive episode. In many cases, the cumulative effects of minor stressful events that occur on a regular basis can be as much of a psychological burden." It can be the daily hassles such as arguments with parents or siblings, they say, that can tip the scales. Perhaps that is why a minor incident, such as being rejected by a romantic interest or not making an athletic team, can cause a teenager to become depressed—or even to attempt suicide.

TRIGGER #8: SEXUAL IDENTITY STRUGGLES. Struggling with an emerging homosexuality is an emotional bombshell. Being gay or lesbian puts the teenager into a sexual minority, making the adolescent struggle to find an identity even more complicated and taxing. Moreover, the world is largely heterosexual and homophobic, and the teen with an emerging homosexuality is often harassed, embarrassed, and even hated.

TRIGGER #9: DIVORCE OR INTENSE MARITAL CONFLICT. Divorcing parents often realize that one or more of their children have become depressed, but doctors aren't sure how divorce may trigger depression. Some say that an event that led up to the divorce—marital conflict or perhaps physical or verbal spousal abuse—is the culprit, not the actual divorce decree. Others, such as Dr. Harold Koplewicz, point to the "cascade" of stressful events that follow: the financial burden of supporting two households, the presence of new suitors or new lovers, or remarriage with a poorly blended family.

TRIGGER #10: DEATH OF A PARENT OR OTHER LOVED ONE. Adolescent grief is no small problem. In the United States, more than 2 million children and adolescents younger than eighteen have experienced the death of a parent. Early adolescents, ages twelve to fourteen, mourn the parent as an adviser, guide, role model, and limit-setter, sometimes even pretending the parent is present and having ongoing conversations with the dead mother or father. Older adolescents are easily overwhelmed by the surviving parent's emotional dependence, concerns, and grief. A teen's grief becomes a marker for depression when there is school refusal, precocious sexual behavior, marked mood swings, withdrawal from peers, or persistence of adultlike grief beyond two months.

TRIGGER #11: CAREGIVING TEENS AND SHADOW SIBLINGS. In an article for the *New York Times,* I wrote about two Chicago teenagers who faced predicaments that can foster depression. Ariceliz Perez is a "parentified" teen who is a caregiver for her developmentally delayed brother, Harry. "I help him in writing and in speaking," she said. "He can't pronounce words very well. He can't say his name right. Sometimes he says his name like 'Hoppy.' I help him tie his shoes and put on his coat. I help him every day after I finish my homework. I watch him on weekends when my mom helps my dad outside cleaning the garage or fixing the car." Maria Cruz, Ariceliz's mother, hasn't missed the point. She said, "She jumps in there. She attends his needs. Actually, Ariceliz is a mother to Harry." Instead of becoming themselves, if the caregiver teen takes on too completely the identity of the parents, this theft of adolescence can promote depression. The other teen, Nathan Weiner, has an autistic brother. Nathan is not parentified, but he is in danger of becoming a "shadow sibling." In families like this, the normal teens may get forgotten at the periphery of the family, because the disabled child occupies the center. Fortunately, Nathan's mother recognizes that this situation is a strong predisposition to depression, and wisely, she has enrolled him in a Chicago support group for teens with disabled siblings.

TRIGGER #12: CHRONIC ILLNESS. A chronic illness may have a dramatic adverse impact on a teenager's psyche. Seizure disorders are especially toxic in this regard. Daily medications, restricted activities, and the stigma of sometimes having to wear a helmet to prevent injury in the event of a major seizure make school a daily ordeal instead of a venue to build self-esteem and social skills. The repeated hospitalizations necessary for cystic fibrosis, the embarrassing need to be near a bathroom with inflammatory bowel disease, the fear of recurrence with childhood cancer, or the isolation with physical handicaps divert precious energy from the tasks of adolescence to painful daily coping.

Has Your Teen Experienced Any of the Triggers for Depression in the Last Year?

Instructions: Circle yes or no for each item.

Trigger #1:	Entering a new school	Yes	No
Trigger #2:	First year of college	Yes	No
Trigger #3:	Too much homework and academic pressure	Yes	No
Trigger #4:	Too many scheduled activities	Yes	No
Trigger #5:	Inadequate social skills or unpopularity	Yes	No
Trigger #6:	Unattractiveness and social rejection	Yes	No
Trigger #7:	Accumulation of small stressors	Yes	No
Trigger #8:	Sexual identity struggles	Yes	No
Trigger #9:	Divorce or intense marital conflict	Yes	No
Trigger #10:	Death of a parent or other loved one	Yes	No
Trigger #11:	Caregiving or "shadow sibling" role	Yes	No
Trigger #12:	Chronic illness	Yes	No

Scoring: Count one point for each yes answer circled, then add up the total.

1 point—The item for which you circled yes merits your careful attention to defuse it right now as a trigger for depression.

Add Up the Clues

2 points—Your teen is on a slippery slope, and you must assess his or her situation periodically. Take all three tests in chapters 3 and 4 every several weeks.

3 or more points—Your teen is ready to tip into depression, and you are now on red alert. Make an appointment for your teen with the family doctor for a formal depression evaluation.

5

Strategy Three
Identify Related Problems— Depression's Companions

Unlike depressed adults, depressed teenagers are likely to come down with a second emotional illness. This co-occurrence is called comorbidity, and only recently have doctors researched this important issue in adolescents. About half of depressed teenagers will simultaneously suffer from a second emotional illness. It's double trouble.

When another emotional illness is heaped onto depression, the consequences are distressing. For one thing, the comorbid illness adversely affects the outcome of the depressive episode. These teens experience a poorer response to antidepressant medications, and they have a greater likelihood of a relapse of the depression.

The comorbid illness also makes certain features of the depression worse, and each illness seems to have a characteristic capacity in this regard. Social anxiety, for example, chips away at self-esteem. ADHD distances the depressed teen even further from peers. The metabolic derangements of the self-inflicted starvation of anorexia nervosa substantially increase the risk of death.

The double suffering these teenagers must endure causes many of them to believe that suicide is an acceptable and attractive alternative to going on this way. Depressed teens with a comorbid emotional illness think about suicide more—and they attempt suicide more. Doctors are beginning to believe that early-onset depression in adolescence, with its high incidence of comorbidity, is a more serious form of the disease.

The high frequency of comorbid emotional illnesses in depressed teens doubles a partnering parent's detective work. Like depression, many of the comorbid illnesses are often not apparent, or they are underdiagnosed. They can occur before, during, or after the start of the depressive episode. Much of the current research, though, indicates that the comorbid illness usually precedes the onset of the depression. This notion is consistent with the theory that depression is often precipitated by some kind of stressor.

As a parental partner, you need look for clues to identify comorbid conditions as diligently as you look for signs of depression. You cannot rely on school counselors, physicians, or therapists to pay sufficient attention to these other problems.

When parents arrive at the doctor's office with their depressed teen, they need to remind the physician about the eight most common comorbid illnesses described below, and request that a clinical assessment be made if there is a suspicion that any of these may coexist with the teen's depression. Conversely, if your teenager does not seem depressed but is afflicted with any of these eight emotional illnesses, you ought to request a formal evaluation for depression.

Generalized Anxiety Disorder

I first suspected that something dark and menacing was growing inside Eric when he was in the eighth grade, a year or so before he slipped into depression. During a "boys' night out" at a spare-ribs restaurant, he unexpectedly burst into tears while we were discussing friendships. "My humor isn't working anymore," he sobbed. This cryptic comment, I only later figured out, meant that he was constantly worrying about his social acceptability. He was trying to entertain peers with humor to compensate for his self-appraised social inadequacy. With a few laughs, he thought, he could make himself acceptable and win them over as friends. He also worried about his adequacy as a student, a tennis player, and a pianist. Although outgoing, charming, and handsome, he was reluctant to form relationships with girls. He shied away from leadership positions at school. Ultimately, he became extremely fidgety, twirled his hair between his thumb and index finger, and chewed his nails until they were stubs. He spoke too fast. Sometimes he gestured wildly with his hands. Often he couldn't sit still. Eric became a nervous wreck.

The anxiety syndrome inflicted a gaping wound on Eric's psyche. When the depression finally came a year later, it tore the wound open even wider. Both illnesses caused Eric to hemorrhage self-worth until he was empty. Eric thought he was nothing but a human-formed shell with nothing whatsoever of value inside. His self-loathing was so great it's no wonder he thought suicide was a reasonable solution.

Eric's experience of having a depression follow on the heels of an anxiety syndrome is sadly typical in depressed teenagers. Scientific studies show that nearly half of depressed adolescents also have generalized anxiety disorder, and that the disorder almost always sets in prior to the depression. Its major features are those of the classic "worrywart," but exaggerated a hundredfold:

- Excessive and pervasive anxiety or worry, especially about issues of competency or adequacy
- Inability to control the worry
- Physical symptoms such as restlessness, easy fatigability, difficulty concentrating, irritability, muscle tension, and sleep disturbances

The Anxiety Disorders Association of America (ADAA) has devised a self-diagnosis test for generalized anxiety disorder. If you are concerned about your teenager's anxiety symptoms, you can gently suggest that he or she check it out on the ADAA Web site (www. adaa.org). This site also offers useful information about symptoms and treatments.

Anorexia Nervosa

The depressed teenager believes she is worthless. The anorexic teen believes she is overweight, even obese. Anorexia thus doubles the depressed teen's distortions in thinking. Worse yet, anorexia adds an extra risk of death. Of all the psychiatric illnesses, anorexia has the highest mortality rate. About 6 percent, maybe even 10 percent, of these young people, mostly women, will die. One-fourth of the deaths will be due to suicide—some consider themselves too fat to live. "It's immediately striking that what you are most afraid of is that you will lose your child," Katie's mother said. "I knew [anorexia] had a mortality rate. The percentage didn't matter. This could be fatal."

Sometimes the anorexia is quite apparent. "With Katie, I saw it coming," her mother said. "My hope was that she was only toying with things and not forming a pattern. Maybe I was denying it. But eventually, I became aware that a process was beginning."

Like depression, anorexia may not announce its presence. "We were totally clueless about her," Alison's stepfather said. "When she was thirteen, she stopped eating with the family. She shopped in the boys' department to buy oversized clothes. Before we figured out what was wrong, she got down to ninety-four pounds and became the 'flier' on her cheerleading squad. That's the person who's so light she gets tossed into the air."

Anorexia nervosa has four telltale signs:

- A refusal to maintain a body weight normal for the child's height and age
- A dread about gaining weight or becoming fat, even though the child is underweight
- An emphasis on body weight as a crucial factor in self-evaluation
- For postpubertal girls, the absence of three consecutive menstrual cycles, since starvation impairs ovarian function

There are two kinds of anorexia. One is the restrictive type, in which the person goes on a program of controlled self-starvation often coupled with compulsive exercising. These people teach themselves to ignore hunger and are adept at pushing food around on their plates with a fork under the guise of eating. Their biggest accomplishment would be, say, to eat only an apple a day.

The second kind of anorexia is the purging type. These anorexics abuse laxatives, diuretics, or enemas and regularly induce vomiting. "Every night after dinner, she would go upstairs to do her homework," Alison's stepfather said. "Little did we know she was going upstairs to throw up. She would keep the window open in her bedroom, even during the winter, to let out the vomit smell. We finally had to take the door off her bedroom."

It's the perfectionist who is most prone to developing anorexia. This kind of personality may have stunted emotional expression and is overly industrious, overly responsible, rigid, and excessively conforming. In fact, group therapy for anorexia can sometimes be counterproductive because the inherent competitiveness of perfectionist personalities may turn the group into contestants who vie with each other to see who can lose the most weight.

In a strange twist, young women have created dozens of Web sites where they share food-deprivation tricks and promote anorexia as a valid lifestyle choice. Although there are many legitimate sources of information about eating disorders online, parents must be careful that cybersurfing teenagers aren't getting the wrong sort of advice from these disturbing pro-anorexia chat rooms and Web sites.

Parents should also be aware that anorexia is no longer the exclusive province of girls. About 10 percent of anorexics are boys. Increasingly, men are basing their attractiveness to the other sex on weight and body shape as hefty earning power is no longer a male prerogative. Moreover, more gay males are developing eating disorders as homosexuality comes out of the closet.

Anorexia used to be thought of as a mental disorder of affluent whites. Not any longer. The values of white culture, which place a premium on thinness, are becoming so pervasive that anorexia is now infecting minorities and lower socioeconomic groups. For many kinds of people, beauty comes only in one size.

The disease is becoming rampant on college campuses. As new college students, teens may for the first time be in control of their own food intake while being independent of parents. And the "freshman fifteen," as Eric says it is called at his college, plagues many incoming students: they often gain ten to fifteen pounds by consuming junk food and large quantities of typical dormitory food high in carbohydrates and fat. Couple this huge calorie intake with the media's insistence that the ideal female form is that of a boy's body with breasts and you have the formula for an epidemic.

Depression can occur before, during, or after the anorexia. Studies show that one-third of anorexics are actually depressed while anorexic. As many as two-thirds of anorexics will ultimately suffer an episode of major depression sometime in their life.

This disease of self-starvation confronts parents with two challenges. The first is to get the teen into treatment. Initially, most anorexics will deny that they have a problem, and parents will have to confront them repeatedly. Even though parental persistence usually succeeds in getting them to their first doctor's appointment, anorexic teens are notorious for not following through with psychiatric treatment because of its stigma.

The second challenge is difficult for parents, because most anorexia has its seeds in troubled family dynamics. Parents may have to come to the uncomfortable realization that the teen's starvation is a symptom of the family's dysfunction. While there are many variations, unhealthy power dynamics within the family seem to be a key factor. In an attempt to get the situation "under control," the girl begins to regulate her eating.

To get the situation into genuine control, parents must take an inventory of themselves. Have courage, and make sure you read chapter 9 on how to do the family inventory. Not only is it essential for your child's depression treatment, but it may be a lifesaver if anorexia is part of the picture.

Obsessive-Compulsive Disorder

Less than two centuries ago, obsessive-compulsive disorder was thought to be caused by demonic possession, and clerics treated it with exorcism. The enlightening discovery that the disorder responds to psychoactive medicines such as Prozac extricates it from the category of Satan's doings and places it squarely in the physiological realm of altered brain circuitry.

This mental illness is rather common in adolescence, especially among boys, and is sometimes called the "hiccups of the mind." This descriptive term emphasizes the persistent and repetitive nature of the behaviors—the compulsions—that the afflicted person feels driven to perform. Some of these compulsive rituals are indeed dramatic, such as excessive hand washing and showering, repetitively walking through the same doorway until it feels "right," or hoarding useless objects such as empty toothpaste tubes.

Why does a person with obsessive-compulsive disorder perform these lengthy or elaborate rituals? One reason is to dispel a particular fear. I must wash my hands every half hour to make sure I don't get infected with those billions of horrible germs that are floating around me. If I don't arrange my shoes precisely the right way, something bad will happen to my family. "Step on a crack, break your mother's back" is a perfect example of an obsession and compulsion if this unwarranted fear repeatedly comes to mind and demands the meticulous stepping of the walker.

A second reason is that the compulsive behaviors are responses to obsessive, but senseless, thoughts. The thoughts are so troubling that compulsive behaviors must be designed to neutralize them. Whenever I'm out driving, I think I may have hit someone and run over his body, so I must look in the rearview mirror every fifteen seconds or so to be sure this horror hasn't happened.

The compulsive actions may also be related to more generalized anxiety and manifested in seemingly inexplicable obsessive behaviors. One fifteen-year-old boy was obsessed with passing through the doorway in his home in a specific manner, and if it didn't feel right to him, he had to walk through the door again and again. One day he passed through the door five hundred times in a row. His alarmed parents finally brought him to a hospital for treatment.

Adolescents with this disorder are usually secretive about their obsessions and compulsions, and they will go to great lengths to disguise them. For example, frequent hand washing may be disguised as bathroom trips for voiding. Or, rituals will be scheduled for secluded "private" time. Parents should be suspicious under certain circumstances:

- Homework, especially, may be a tip-off. Teenagers with obsessive-compulsive disorder may get bogged down in homework. They may be unable to complete an assignment because their handwriting must be just so, paragraphs must be reread incessantly, or a math problem must be solved repeatedly because the last solution wasn't quite right. Some teens will actually erase and re-erase their homework until they make holes in the paper.
- A preoccupation with germs and contamination.
- Peculiar ordering, arranging, or hoarding behaviors.
- Elaborate bedtime rituals such as getting in the bed on a certain side or repeating "good night" in a proscribed way.
- The teen may repeatedly remark that he has an "overactive imagination."

Obsessive-compulsive disorder makes depression worse. The depressed teen is brooding about real-life problems such as self-worth, friendships, or hope. Combine the recurring thoughts of obsessive-compulsive disorder with the rumination of depression and you double the amount of brooding. This kind of teenager wonders if he is going mad, because he is drowning in a torrent of toxic thoughts.

Since teens tend to underreport their obsessions and compulsions to parents or doctors, parents must be keenly observant and take the lead if they suspect symptoms. As a first step, they can ask their teenager to log on to the Web site of the Anxiety Disorders

Association of America (www.adaa.org) and take an obsessive-compulsive-disorder self-diagnosis test. A copy of the test results should be taken to the appointment with the teen's primary care physician. The psychiatric evaluation of this kind of comorbid teen can be complex, and so parents should not hesitate to request a referral to a mental health specialist.

Oppositional-Defiant Disorder

Can behavior typical of the "terrible twos" reemerge in the teen years? Sadly, yes. When it's extreme, psychiatrists call it oppositional-defiant disorder.

A teenager with this mental illness habitually displays negativistic and defiant behavior, refusing to conform to the ordinary requirements of authority figures such as parents or teachers. This is the truly hostile teenager who talks back, ignores homework, continually "forgets" things, refuses to keep a tidy room, and always procrastinates. The lack of compliance can be so great that parents think the teenager is hard of hearing and will take her to a physician to have her ears checked. Her personality traits are far from charming. She often loses her temper and is argumentative, touchy, resentful, stubborn, spiteful, and deliberately annoying.

What makes oppositional-defiant disorder even more annoying is that the ill teenager often defies authority by passive or covert means. "She would do things just to piss us off," Michelle's father said. "We didn't like rap music, so she would play rap music to stuff it down our throats. We didn't allow her to drink, but she would leave a vodka bottle out on the counter for us to find."

When many of us were teenagers, we occasionally displayed some of this kind of obnoxious behavior. After all, learning to resist the will of others, or even oppose it, is a normal part of maturation.

It's important for parents to understand the difference between annoying but normal behavior and the symptoms of oppositional-defiant disorder.

For a psychiatrist to consider this kind of behavior a genuine mental disorder, it must pass at least two tests. First, the pattern of behavior must be present for a minimum of six months. Second, the behavior disturbance must cause significant impairment in the teen's ability to get along at school, with friends, or on the job.

Oppositional-defiant disorder is a particularly unfortunate addition to depression because it usually robs the teenager of her best adult helpers, her parents. "We were ready to throw her out of the house," Michelle's father said. "There were many times I just stayed at work with a book and read. I couldn't come home. I wanted to escape."

If this kind of teenager readily alienates parents, who else can help? Michelle's father wisely recognized the invaluable role of grandparents. "If there was one thing her grandfather was proud of, it was his grandparenting. She and her grandfather had long talks when she felt she wasn't getting much solace out of us." Parents may also have to recruit teachers, clergy, an influential coach, or a favorite aunt or uncle, just as Dr. Cheryl King does with the Youth Nominated Support Team.

Attention-Deficit/Hyperactivity Disorder (ADHD)

Young Jared had an explosive personality. "He might as well have had a sign pinned to his back that said, 'Pick on me—I can't take it,' " his mother said.

Jared had all the classic signs of ADHD in kindergarten— inattention, hyperactivity, and impulsivity with regard to rule-governed behavior. "I decided to do a videotape of Jared at school when he was five to see what he was doing all day," his mother said. "I went home crying. He jumped from group to group every several minutes. It was my awakening. It went downhill from there. In the third grade, his teachers locked him in a room by himself. He had gotten into a fight on the playground. That was the same year a teacher put red Magic Marker dots on his nose and made him stand in front of the class because he wouldn't sit still." Jared was typical of children with ADHD. He was driven, restless, and never tired. And for all of his "effort," he produced little.

When Jared became a teenager, his self-esteem plummeted even more, and he became significantly depressed. "Jared's ADHD and depression were interconnected," his mother said. "He was rejected from friendships. He was rejected by his cousins. And he was rejected by church youth groups. There was no place for him to step out. So he withdrew. He spent most of his time in his bedroom because he wasn't spending time with other kids. He was stuck on the computer, stuck on solitaire, and stuck on TV news."

That is precisely how ADHD makes depression worse. Depression forces many teens to withdraw, erecting around themselves nearly impenetrable barriers from which they can seldom escape. Even if they do venture out, because of the impulsivity of ADHD, they often meet a crowd of disapproving peers who don't want to associate with them. ADHD coupled with depression can make the isolation and loneliness unbearable.

ADHD is now frequently diagnosed—and some would argue overdiagnosed—in young children by school counselors. By the teen years, most parents of ADHD kids are already well aware of the problem. What's important to recognize as a parental detective is the link between ADHD and depression. The child whose self-esteem has already been battered by ADHD is especially vulnerable to the feelings of hopelessness and worthlessness spawned by depression.

Substance Abuse

Although the rates of teenage drug use and drug abuse appear to be declining recently, they remain stubbornly high. A survey of thousands of teens by Partnership for a Drug-Free America, a coalition of communications professionals, found that 40 percent said they had tried marijuana at some point, and 10 percent said they had used ecstasy. About 20 percent had used dangerous volatile inhalants such as gasoline, butane, paint thinner, spot removers, and whipped-cream propellant. Smaller but still significant numbers of teenagers use or abuse cocaine, hallucinogens, psychoactive prescription drugs such as painkillers or tranquilizers, and even nonprescription drugs such as stimulant-laden cold remedies.

Although illegal for underage adolescents, alcohol is still the legal drug they abuse the most. Scientists at Columbia University have calculated that American underage drinkers consume an astonishing 20 billion drinks per year. Teenage drinking rates have hardly declined in the past decade, and 5 million teenagers admit to binge drinking at least once a month. An unfortunate trend is that the age at which our children begin drinking is getting younger, and a third of the teenagers who drink say they started in the eighth grade or earlier. Experts worry that the developing brain of teenagers makes them more prone to addiction. Although teenagers are bombarded with ads about the dangers of drinking, teenage TV characters are shown with alcohol more often than with any other beverage. An overworked father, a stressed-out mother, or a derelict are the usual images of the alcoholic that our mind conjures up. We forget that the cute eleventh-grader who is a cheerleader and manages to get passing grades but binges on beer every weekend is also a valid image of someone hooked on alcohol.

Depression puts a teenager at increased risk for developing a drug abuse problem. In fact, about a third of depressed teens will have a concurrent drug or alcohol problem, and studies show that most of the time the addiction followed the onset of the depression. This supports the notion that the addiction to alcohol or some other "feel-good" substance represents the teen's attempt at self-medication. The teen tries the substance to see if it will diminish the emotional pain of depression, finds out that indeed it does, and then goes on to use it regularly for relief. Especially at risk are depressed teens with physical disabilities that cause them to be excluded from peer activities. Depressed gay and lesbian teens are at risk for alcohol abuse to blunt the feelings of guilt or inadequacy, because 80 percent of them are teased or bullied in their schools or communities.

The combination of depression and substance abuse makes for a substantially worse prognosis. For a teenager who is also addicted, the depressive episode usually is deeper, responds less favorably to antidepressant medications, and has a greater chance of recurrence. Postmortem tests of depressed teens who commit suicide show that about half the time alcohol or an illicit drug was a contributing factor.

There are significant barriers to getting treatment for teen drug or alcohol abuse. Addicted teens, like addicted adults, will deny they have any sort of problem, and parents will sometimes legitimize the teen's denial with trivializing comments like "It's only booze or pot—it's no big deal." Remember, just because you might have indulged in high school or college doesn't mean that drugs and alcohol are harmless fun for teenagers. The potential for addiction, drunk-driving accidents, and overdoses is too serious to take lightly.

According to pediatricians, substance abuse may be the single most frequently missed diagnosis in adolescents. About the only way a doctor encounters a teenager with a clear-cut substance-abuse problem is in the emergency room with an overdose, or with a serious injury related to the substance. Otherwise, addicted teens just don't show up in a doctor's office with the easily distinguishable signs and symptoms of substance abuse. Pediatricians ought to maintain a high index of suspicion, but they frankly admit they could do a much better job. As a rule, they get little formal substance-abuse training in their residencies. Many of them feel uncomfortable broaching the issue or treating addiction problems. Some of them relate poorly to teenagers, getting stuck in the mode of being the "baby doctor." And truncated appointment time and inadequate third-party reimbursement may preclude their discussing substance abuse during an office visit.

The facts are clear. The parent must maintain the index of suspicion and be alert to a few clues:

1. The teen shows behavior changes such as marked mood swings, worrisome risk-taking, or promiscuity. The teen may also be stealing to buy otherwise unaffordable drugs.
2. Academic performance may deteriorate. The teen skips classes or entire school days. Judgment or memory are impaired. Grades fall, and disciplinary difficulties with teachers may sometimes occur, resulting in suspension or expulsion.
3. New and peculiar personal habits evolve. The teen loses interest in sports or develops new friends. Dress and music interests change, and the teen may pay less attention to personal hygiene.
4. Physical symptoms start to show: red eyes, nasal stuffiness and irritation, unremitting cough, hoarseness, or physical injuries due to episodes of intoxication.

If any of these get your attention, the next step is to confront your teenager with your worries—and gently, because an addicted teen will be defensive. The first confrontation may be unproductive, and you may have to revisit the issue the next day or the next week. Persistence is key. Dr. Francis Mondimore, a Johns Hopkins psychiatrist, warns about depressed and addicted teens that "patients who do not get treatment for both problems will not recover from either."

Make an appointment with the teen's doctor and alert the doctor beforehand about the reason you are coming. Don't necessarily expect a toxicology screen. Although some psychiatrists recommend obtaining a urine sample from any teenager who shows emotional symptoms, the results of such screens seem hit-and-miss owing to the nature of the drug and the time it was last used. Also don't necessarily expect the doctor to administer one of those sophisticated questionnaires such as the Substance Abuse Subtle Screening Inventory (SASSI). Many doctors, and many studies, insist that person-to-person directness is the most effective way of detecting substance abuse. Doing so, however, requires a skilled, motivated, and non-judgmental doctor—who also is optimistic about the value of substance-abuse treatment. If your child's doctor does not meet these requirements, find a new doctor.

Right now, about one of every eight American children has a parent with a current or previous drinking problem. These children of alcoholic parents are at great risk—they are about five times more likely to become alcoholics than other children. It may be genetic. It may also be the family environment, because alcoholic families typically have problems with feeling, trusting, or communicating. The home may be a place of emotional chaos, poor communication, verbal or physical abuse, neglect, or parental fighting. Alcoholic parents may be so wrapped up in their own problems that they have little time left over for the teenager's. It's no wonder then that the teen would turn to alcohol or some other substance to ease the pain and find a refuge. If you as a parent feel you have an addiction, the realization of your child's depression ought to serve as your wake-up call. You can't really help your child recover from the depression if you don't recover from your addiction. Worse yet, your addiction may be contributing to your child's depression. Make sure you read chapter 9 in this book on taking the family inventory and finding help with issues that come to light.

Dysthymia

This is an especially pernicious kind of low-mood disorder. Dr. Neal Ryan, a psychiatrist at the University of Pittsburgh, says, "It's a horrible disease with a horrible course." Dysthymia is a cloudy day, all day and every day. It's a low-grade funk that lasts for at least a year. It's no consolation that the depressive symptoms are less severe, because the special danger of dysthymia is that the pessimistic and gloomy mood can become chronic and may even last for your teen's entire life. This malicious depressive fog is not so dense, but it is pervasive and persistent. Family, friends, jobs, vacations—everything becomes bland and muted, and for years.

Dysthymic teenagers are unattractively irritable and self-deprecating. It's no surprise, then, that they are often dismissed by their peers as peculiar sad-sack people it would be better not to date or invite to parties. Worse yet, at least 70 percent of dysthymic teens will eventually experience an episode of major depression, a combination ominously named double depression. Mental health scientists at the Oregon Institute have discovered that the episode of major depression usually occurs within three years of the onset of the dysthymia.

Go back now to page 60 and review the symptoms of depression. If you think your teen has been suffering with one or both of the core symptoms for about a year, but you don't judge the symptoms as too severe, and if you think your teen has only two of the additional symptoms, he may be suffering from dysthymia. Get help now and ward off a major depressive episode that may be on the horizon.

Mania and Bipolar Disorder

Mania frightens parents. A manic episode is officially defined as a distinct period of abnormally and persistently elevated, expansive, or irritable mood. To qualify as a genuine manic episode it should be severe enough to require hospitalization or cause marked impairment in functioning at school, in the family, or on the job. It lasts at least a week. Moreover, your teen must show at least three or four of the following symptoms:

- Delusions of grandeur or inflated self-esteem
- Flight of ideas, or the teen admitting that "my thoughts are racing"
- Decreased need for sleep—for example, feeling rested after only three or four hours of sleep
- More talkative than usual—talking "binges" or pressure to keep talking
- Increased goal-directed activity, either socially or at school
- Distractibility, with the teen's attention too easily drawn to unimportant or irrelevant matters
- Excessive involvement in pleasurable activities that have a high potential for painful consequences, such as buying sprees or sexual indiscretions

The week of mania may be pure and constant mania, or it may be punctuated by a few depressive-like symptoms. When this kind of severe mania precedes or follows a depressive episode, psychiatrists call it bipolar I disorder. When the manic episode is less severe—it lasts four days or less and does not require hospitalization or result in significant impairment—it is called hypomanic. The combination of hypomanic episodes and depressive episodes is called bipolar II disorder.

Bipolar disorder used to be called manic depression and was viewed as the exclusive domain of unfortunate adults such as

Ernest Hemingway. But now doctors are saying that in a single generation the average age of onset of bipolar disorder has mysteriously fallen from the early thirties to the late teens. Grunge-rock musician Kurt Cobain, for example, suffered from bipolar disorder from adolescence. He self-medicated with alcohol and other drugs and eventually took his own life before he turned thirty. Unfortunately, Cobain's tragic life illustrates that bipolar disorder must be diagnosed promptly and treated vigorously. It's not just the torment. Victims have an alcoholism and drug-abuse rate three times the average. Some doctors put their suicide rate as high as 20 percent.

About half of adults claim their bipolar symptoms began before or during adolescence. Many of these adults were not diagnosed as teens and waited up to ten years before their condition was recognized and treatment was instituted. As a parent, you cannot afford to miss the obvious warning signs:

- Your teenager may already have been diagnosed with depression, but she seems to "cycle" between highs and lows—and this can happen even every couple of hours or days. You shouldn't necessarily find relief in her frequent and rapid reversions to a good mood. The mood may be too good, and it may qualify as mania.
- A diagnosis of ADHD sometimes is incorrect. The child's hyperactivity is wrongly ascribed to this condition when actually the frenetic behavior is mania. (In fact, Cobain's first diagnosis as a teenager was ADHD, and this might have been off the mark.) What may seem to be ADHD and depression may actually be bipolar disorder.
- Beverages containing caffeine—coffee, tea, cola, and certain other soft drinks—trigger not just nervousness but extreme hyperactivity.
- A close relative has bipolar disorder—and your teenager seems manic or hypomanic.

Bipolar disorder is a debilitating disease, but one that can be controlled with modern medicines. Carrie Fisher, the Princess Leia of *Star Wars* fame, has testified to that happy outcome on several talk shows. She couldn't escape some of its ravages, but she learned to manage her condition well and works regularly in Hollywood as a superb "script doctor."

To find out more about this potentially devastating teen illness, log on to the Web site of the Child & Adolescent Bipolar Foundation (www.bpkids.org).

The Ten Parental Partnering Strategies and the Comorbid Disorders

It's beyond the scope of this book to provide comprehensive discussions of the symptoms, causes, and treatments for each of the comorbid disorders. Each condition is worthy of an entire book on the subject—and many have been written. The goal here is to ensure that you, as the parental partner, look for warning signs in your teenager and advocate for accurate diagnosis and appropriate treatment.

Existence of a comorbid disorder often requires steps beyond the strategies outlined in this book. For example, treatment of anorexia or substance abuse may entail a stay at a hospital or detoxification center. Comorbid disorders also need to be considered when medication for depression is prescribed. It can be disastrous for a depressed teen with manic episodes or a drug addiction to be arbitrarily prescribed a dose of Prozac or Zoloft for depression by a general practitioner. In these cases, medications must be carefully prescribed and monitored by a specialist.

The good news is that the Strategies of Parental Partnering will serve double duty if your teenager has a comorbid disorder. The steps you take to rescue your teenager from depression will also help you and your child manage the additional problem—particularly if you're aware of the condition and incorporate it into the strategies from the onset. That's why being a detective and presenting your findings to the doctor and therapist is crucial. A coherent view of the whole picture will enable you and the health-care team to customize medications and treatment programs for the best possible outcome.

6

Strategy Four
Be Alert—Suicide Risk and Prevention

It was four o'clock in the morning, and Dan's unnerved and disbelieving mother sat on the living room sofa rereading her fifteen-year-old son's suicide note. "I must have read it ten times that night," she said. A few hours earlier Dan had hysterically rushed into his mother's bedroom. He shook her awake and sobbed, "I don't want to die, Mom. I don't want to die." Dan was now sleeping peacefully on the sofa, his head nestled on her lap, just as he used to when he was a little boy. He had taken an overdose of trazodone, an antidepressant medication. "The doctors and the people at the poison control center told me that the number of pills he took wouldn't harm him, but he would sleep for several days," his mother said. "I understood he was depressed, but he never talked about death, or suicide, or anything terribly dark." Dan's mother continued to study the "brutal" four-page letter, looking for any clues that he might try it again. Perhaps his next attempt would be fatal.

Suicides are always calamities, especially those of our teenagers, because they die so young. Schopenhauer said that when the terrors of life outweigh the terrors of death, a person will likely put an end to himself. How shocking it is when a young person loses hope that the terrors will subside and life will have promise.

Doctors in the United States became increasingly alarmed about adolescent suicide during the last half of the twentieth century, because the rate was steadily climbing. In 1998, 4,153 young persons aged fifteen to twenty-four took their own lives. Now, thank God, the rate is starting to decrease. In 2000, 3,877 young people committed suicide. Still, this means that about every two hours an adolescent considers life so hopeless that a reasonable and welcome solution is self-slaughter.

An astonishing 19.3 percent of adolescents admit to serious thoughts about suicide, according to the 2001 Youth Risk Behavior Survey conducted by the Centers for Disease Control and Prevention (CDC). No one is quite sure why the percentage is so high. One reason, perhaps, is that high school is no longer a nurturing place, the kind idyllically portrayed in *Happy Days*. Instead, high school is fraught with pressures, from academic to sexual. Others indict the modern tendency to devalue the family. And some doctors are quick to point out that adults nowadays subject teens to much more stress by turning up the pressure to excel at school, or by overbooking their schedules. The CDC's survey paints a frightening picture of unhappy youth and went on to show that suicide ideation in many of these teens had worrisomely progressed to more concrete stages—15 percent were putting together a suicide plan, and 8.8 percent had made an actual suicide attempt, with one-third of the attempts being dangerous enough to require medical attention.

When Eric told me, "Dad, now I understand why people kill

themselves," he got my immediate attention. Hurting badly, he was worried about himself enough to admit his suicide ideation. Some ideation is more "fanciful" than Eric's—if that is ever an acceptable word to be used about suicidal thoughts. For example, Alison's stepfather said, "She would lock herself in the bathroom and shout through the door that she was going to drink all the Drano under the sink. Fifteen minutes later she would be downstairs wrapped up watching TV." Another depressed teenager, Matthew, would threaten to slash his wrists with a ballpoint pen.

Some ideas about suicide are silent, made known only by the actual attempt. That was the case for both Dan and Lauren. Lauren's mother was completely taken by surprise when she heard that her daughter had jumped off a second-story deck, the first of three suicide attempts that Lauren would make in high school.

I felt relieved that Eric would confide his thoughts to me. I also felt fortunate, even blessed, to get this alert before he did anything catastrophic. The alert is no less meaningful when the ideation is fanciful. You should consider the alert flashing brightly purely because your teen is depressed: fully 90 percent of young people who commit suicide suffer from an emotional illness, usually a mood disorder such as depression, and psychiatrists at Cornell University think even this percentage is an underestimate. Because Eric was depressed, I needed to figure out how intense and frequent Eric's ideation was. This was not an overreaction. Studies of depressed teenagers show that they commit suicide even when the depression is moderate rather than severe, and even when the depression has only been of short duration. Moreover, the youngest teenagers will make the fewest suicide "comments" before they actually attempt it. I couldn't afford to get lulled into complacency just because his talk about it was casual and infrequent.

As a parental partner, you need to undertake six steps to prevent suicide. Each step is difficult. Each step may save your son's or your daughter's life.

Step 1—Assess how strongly your teenager might be thinking about suicide.

Broach the subject as soon as you realize your teen is depressed. Most of all, trust your instincts. You know your teenager best.

Psychiatrists and psychologists have devised questionnaire-type inventories with formal scoring systems that they use in their offices to assess the severity of the ideation. At home, you can make a fairly good estimate of how intense and frequent the thoughts are simply by talking to your teenager. The kinds of answers you get will tell you how alarmed you ought to be. The best approach is to be direct. "I know you are down in the dumps. Have you ever thought about hurting yourself?" If directness is not for you or your teen, then try the side door. "Kurt Cobain killed himself. What do you or your friends think about that?" If you are rebuffed because that tactic turned out to be transparent, admit it—but persist nevertheless. "I'm your parent, and I'm worried about you. What do you think about suicide?" Be sure you show your genuine concern even when your teenager is angry or rageful.

If you can engage your teenager in this kind of conversation, these are some specific items you need to address:

- *Presence of suicidal thoughts*—How frequently does your teenager have them? How long do the thoughts last—a minute, an hour, all day, never go away?
- *Attitude toward suicide*—Does your teen consider it a good idea? Is it a betrayal of your teenager's values or a violation of his religious beliefs? Does he think his family or friends would be better off without him because he is a burden?
- *The specific reason for the suicidal thoughts*—Does your teenager feel like a failure at school, work, or among friends? Does life seem

hopeless or too much work to be worthwhile? Has your teen been disappointed by others?

- *Suicide plan*—Has your teenager chosen a method (for example, a firearm or an overdose) and assessed its availability? Has your teenager begun to put the plan in motion or given away valued possessions? Has your teen formed a suicide pact with other teens?
- *Suicide note or letter*—Has your teen thought about what it should contain or actually begun composing one?

Step 2—Snoop if necessary.

Yes, I'm serious. When your teenager refuses to talk about suicide or gives you incomplete, evasive, or untruthful answers, there is no alternative. The stakes are too high. Don't forget that teenage boys have particular difficulty in talking about emotional pain.

So, you don't like the idea of spying on your teenager? Consider this. If you suspected your daughter had an eating disorder, would you go through her drawers and medicine cabinet to look for laxatives? If you thought your son was using heroin or crack, would you search his room for drugs and drug paraphernalia? Almost every parent would answer yes—and almost every adolescent psychologist would agree—because the purpose is to save a teen's life. And so it is also with depression. The stakes are too high not to seriously consider this alternative. Both Lauren and Dan made suicide attempts without ever hinting about their intentions to their parents.

Even if your teenager seems willing to talk, consider that lying to parents is part of a teen's way of life. "He had lied to me about going to class the day before he took his life," Frank's mother said. "He was lying about studying, relationships, and drinking and driving. He hung himself in our basement. I found him and cut him down to try to give him CPR." Blake's mother said, "We made a verbal contract after his first suicide attempt that he would never try it again. He went into his bedroom and shot himself. Maybe he was lying."

Still, you should carefully weigh the choice to snoop. Your purpose must be to gather potentially lifesaving information, not to satisfy your curiosity about unrelated aspects of your teenager's lifestyle. You must also be willing to take the heat if your teenager discovers that you're snooping. It may cause a huge blowout, righteous indignation on the part of your teenager, more resentment and less trust. But if it saves your child's life, it's justified—and well worth the temporary rift.

There are four effective ways to snoop.

Talk to your teenager's teachers, coaches, counselors, and friends' parents. I didn't do this for Eric, and that turned out to be a big mistake. Several of Eric's teachers and counselors were suspicious that he was depressed, and they approached him about it when he was a sophomore in high school. However, they never contacted me, and I should have taken the initiative and told them of my concerns. And three years after Eric's depression, one of his friends' mother told me, "Peter knew all along that Eric was struggling." All of these people had valuable information about Eric's depression and suicide risk—and I had never tapped into it.

Monitor your teen's Internet usage. Just do an Internet search on how to commit suicide and see the terrifying things you turn up. Companies such as SecuritySoft and SpectorSoft make snooping software for parents that let you monitor a teen's e-mail, chat rooms, instant messages, message board postings, visited Web sites, and even their passwords. This software will e-mail you a report instantly, hourly, or at a specified time. You can create key phrases such as "suicide," "overdose," or "kill myself," and the software will alert you to all material containing them. Other companies such as WebRoot and Watch Right make software that does not have remote monitoring capability. Instead, their software requires you to log on from the computer your teen uses, which can be a trickier proposition. Another alternative is to use the parental controls that come free with AOL and MSN, which are far from comprehensive but will give you a general idea of what your teenager is doing at the computer. If you have misgivings about snooping software, then, please, at least make a rule that your teenager can use the computer only when the door to his room is open.

Search your teenager's room. "Lauren would burn herself with butane lighters," her mother said. "Once she even heated up an earring with a lighter and branded her arm with it. She was cutting herself with knives she took from the kitchen. I always went through her drawers for lighters and knives." Besides lethal means such as firearms and pills, you should search for drugs and alcohol. These substances make teens impulsive, and teenage suicide is an impulsive act. Of course you may turn up nothing, because teens are clever at hiding. I searched Eric's room for evidence of alcohol but never found anything because he was crushing the beer cans flat and sneaking them out in his backpack with his books the next morning.

Read your teenager's journal or diary. "I could gauge her suicide risk by how her diary read," Lauren's mother said. "A special tip-off was her poetry and how dark it was. She felt she was a worthless person. I thought it was okay because she left her diary out like she wanted me to find it. If she had hidden it, I would go find it. It's a matter of life and death, and doggone it, I'm looking for it. I didn't feel guilty because I was protecting her."

Online Help

An excellent resource for evaluating suicide ideation and risk is Columbia University's TeenScreen. It is in a pilot stage now, but this program offers teens a self-administered, computerized suicide screening test at over sixty high schools in twenty-eight states. If the test reveals a significant risk, a mental health professional interviews the teen. Parents get a report of all results. By the time this book is published, the test should be available online at www.teenscreen.org. Also, the National Alliance for the Mentally Ill has published a Web page about teen suicide (www.nami.org/helpline/teensuicide). Insist that your teen read it. It might spark a discussion.

Step 3—If you judge your teen's thoughts about suicide to be serious, take immediate action at home to decrease the suicide risk.

Some thoughts about suicide are mere fancy. Matthew's father rightly judged Matthew's talk about slashing his wrists with a ballpoint pen as purely fanciful. Some psychiatrists also speak of the "free-floating" idea of suicide—the thought that occasionally comes to mind, but is never entertained as a genuine option. For example, students faced with a particularly fearsome exam are sometimes known to take time out from their study group to discuss with each other various ways of committing suicide should they fail the test. The purpose of the conversation is strictly to entertain each other and, perhaps, to vent some anxiety. After a gruesome and sometimes laughter-filled discussion, though, they get back to studying and forget the discussion ever happened. However, even the slightest grade above these kinds of fanciful thoughts ought to be considered serious. Then you should do the following.

Make sure your depressed teenager is taking antidepressant medications. Although researchers aren't certain, one of the more plausible explanations for the recent decrease in teen suicide rates is that doctors are prescribing antidepressants much more frequently. Keep watch to see if your teen is showing a benefit from the drugs. If not, contact your family physician and, if necessary, request switching to a different drug. You are a partner with the physician. Don't be afraid to say, "This isn't working. We must try something else." Details on evaluating the benefits and side effects of drugs are in chapter 7.

Remove lethal means from the house. This is called "sanitizing" the house. Five times more adolescent boys complete suicide than girls, and they usually choose violent means such as firearms. Rid the house of all firearms and ammunition. Adolescent girls make more suicide attempts than boys, and they often try it with a drug overdose. Check medicine cabinets for drugs that could be injurious or lethal in overdoses. Establish yourself as the custodian of all your teen's medications, doling them out only as needed. If your teenager might prefer a different lethal means, address that also. "Lauren liked to cut herself because she could feel the anger being released," her mother said. "I always kept good count of the kitchen knives and where they were."

Address the drug and alcohol problem right now. Of the people who succeed in committing suicide, more are intoxicated than not. Both drugs and alcohol decrease judgment and increase impulsiveness, and teenage suicide is an impulsive act. "Dan never said to me that he was thinking about this for a long time," his mother said. On the spur of the moment one night, an overdose seemed like the best thing to do.

Address family dysfunction without delay. Much teenage depression is promoted by family dysfunction and instability, with parental addictions, abuse, and parent-child conflict ranking high. The speed and quality of the resolution of the teen's depression is often directly related to solving the family's problems. Make sure to read chapter 9 on the family inventory—and take the appropriate action right away.

Talk to your teen about self-criticism. Numerous studies link suicide to hopelessness, and hopelessness seems to be a constant motive mentioned by those teens who attempt suicide. Be sure to select a therapist who will address your teenager's self-criticism, and use the techniques in chapter 10 to continue the therapeutic work at home.

Start an insomnia watch. Night changes everything. You probably know from personal experience that the thought of an overdue bill at two o'clock in the afternoon is merely a nagging nuisance. At two in the morning, however, you wonder if it will lead to a repossession or even a court appearance. Depression causes insomnia in many teens, and those late wakeful hours are prime time for the kind of self-loathing that seems to justify suicide. (Unfortunately, one of the side effects of some antidepressants is insomnia.) I kept an insomnia watch for Eric. I would monitor whether the lights or the TV or the computer screen were on in his room during the late-night hours. If so, I would invite him downstairs to watch a cheerful movie depicting "people liking people" or just sit in his room and talk about "good" things such as his accomplishments or his plans for the future. Like most depressed teens, Eric tended to remember only negative life events. He even viewed neutral events as negative. He desperately needed some midnight sun. Eric later admitted to me that the darkest hours of the night were the darkest hours of his soul.

Step 4—Notify a health-care professional that your teenager has thought about suicide.

If your teenager is already seeing a mental health therapist, you're still responsible for notifying that person of the suicide ideas. Don't assume the therapist knows already, and that you are only second in line to discover it. While conducting the interviews for this book, I was surprised to find out how often teenagers were dissatisfied with their therapist. Many of them worried about a breach of confidentiality, too. This combination makes for poor communication. A parent may have significantly better rapport and powers of discovery for an issue as sensitive and charged as ending one's life. You may also be frightened about how severe the suicide risk appears. For example, your teen may already have formulated a workable plan. Or, your teen may have ceased functioning and locked himself away in his room, as Blake did the week before he took his own life. It is up to you to ask if an urgent hospitalization is necessary. Trust the wisdom of your parental intuition, and don't be intimidated by professionals. If you believe a hospitalization is necessary, be a proactive partner and push for it.

If your depressed teenager is not seeing any kind of therapist, now is the time to pick up the phone and notify your family doctor that your child is in real danger of committing suicide. Treatment will thus begin, and it could be a lifesaver. Moreover, give your family doctor all your reasons for believing that the risk of suicide is genuine. He can use this information with your insurer as evidence to justify starting or extending mental health benefits.

You may have no family doctor—or no health insurance. This doesn't make your task impossible, only a bit more difficult and inconvenient. A fact of medical practice these days is that your local hospital's emergency room has evolved into a psychiatric crisis center and psychiatric walk-in clinic. So, use it as it's come to be—a good and handy resource, ready twenty-four hours a day. All you need to do is show up. Doctors there will be able to jump-start your teenager's needed entry into the mental health care system, and enterprising social workers may even be able to find state or federal benefits to cover the cost of extended treatment.

Step 5—Assess your teen's situation for any factors that could escalate the suicidal thoughts into suicidal action.

Doctors have interviewed thousands of teenagers who have made suicide attempts. Their interviews point out crucial factors that could put a teenager over the brink from just thinking about suicide to actually attempting it. If any of the factors below applies, put yourself on an especially heightened alert for a possible attempt, even if your estimate of the suicidal ideation is low. These factors elevate the risk for suicide.

Isolation from parents. Isolation can magnify the depressed teen's notion of worthlessness. The teen may be isolated from her parents because they have rejected her, or simply because they are distracted or too busy for her. Worse, the isolation may be the result of physical, sexual, or verbal abuse. Not only is the abused teenager alienated from one or both parents, but she is also denied opportunities in the home for developing the necessary social skills for healthy, nonantagonistic relationships with others. The isolation doubles, then, because she becomes alienated from important adults outside the home such as teachers or coaches. When a depressed teen decides to live away from both parents, the problem is less an intensification of the worthlessness but rather lack of access to the invaluable day-to-day support parents provide. Depressed teens find themselves in this dangerous situation, without a safety net, when they run away from home or get their own apartment and a job after leaving school. Even going away to live at college with their parents' blessing can be perilous.

Being a victim of homophobia. It's been fifteen years since a government report suggested that gay teenagers were at an increased risk for suicide. Being gay, lesbian, bisexual, or transgendered often makes the teen the target of prejudice. Prejudice damages the psyche. Worse yet, if the person is depressed, it intensifies any ongoing sense of worthlessness. The Safe Schools Coalition estimated that in my home state of Minnesota up to 31 percent of gay, lesbian, and bisexual students had attempted suicide. It was perhaps the biggest factor in Dan's tenth-grade attempt, especially since he had an early sexual debut. "There had been a huge incident at school," his mother said. "Boys had encircled him and called him, 'Faggot, faggot.' At that point, he was ostracized." Dan was taunted mercilessly at school, but one-third of students who are struggling with sexual identity get even worse treatment by being physically harassed, sometimes with a weapon. In fact, sixteen-year-old Fred Martinez was bludgeoned to death in Colorado for choosing to live his life as a girl. Your teenager may be questioning his sexuality, or maybe he's gone beyond the questioning stage but is not disclosing it. If you are uncomfortable bringing up the subject, you can get some valuable tips on how to start the conversation and keep it going by reading the National Mental Health Association's pamphlet "What Does Gay Mean?" You can obtain it free of charge online at www.nmha .org/whatdoesgaymean. Other must-visit Web sites are those of the Gay, Lesbian, and Straight Education Network (www.glsen.org) and Parents, Families, and Friends of Lesbians and Gays (www .pflag.org).

Alienation from peers. You don't have to be gay to be bullied, and gangs of bullies aren't always boys. Girl bullies are called queen bees, alpha girls, or RMGs (really mean girls) says Rachel Simmons, author of *Odd Girl Out: The Hidden Culture of Aggression in Girls.* She says girls engage in "alternative aggression." They don't do the boys' shove or punch type. Rather, they circulate "petitions" to hate someone, carry on cruel whispering campaigns, or just refuse to talk to a certain girl. The isolation can be so complete that it spells alienation. About one-third of teenage girls will admit to being bullied, and victims are often depressed, develop eating disorders, or harbor suicidal thoughts. Girls now classify bullying as a more prevalent and agonizing problem than pressure to have sex. Erika Harold, Miss America 2003, was taunted as a ninth-grader with slurs like *whore* and *slut*. She has pleaded that parents be "advocates for their children when they are victimized." Unfortunately, school administrators may turn a deaf ear to your concerns. Alternative aggression is a new concept that many of them are having trouble coming to grips with or are even denying.

Serious conflict outside the home. Being disenfranchised from school, the hub of adolescent life, increases a teen's risk for suicide. The loss of connectedness to school usually results from some type of serious conflict there—habitual disciplinary problems, suspensions and expulsions, or severe academic underperformance with unmet school goals. All of these scenarios lead to dropping out, and new studies show that potential or actual school dropouts are more prone to attempting suicide. Conflicts with the police and subsequent involvement in the judicial system usually result from antisocial behavior, what used to be called juvenile delinquency. Today, psychiatrists call it conduct disorder—persistent aggressive and destructive behavior encompassing such things as stealing, vandalism, truancy, curfew violations, fighting, physical cruelty, and forced sexual activity. The danger here is grave, since studies now show that about one-third of teenage boys who commit suicide have a conduct disorder. All these kinds of conflicts have one common theme—alienation of the teenager from adult social systems outside the home. As a parent, you may be the only person who hasn't given up on him.

Certain comorbid conditions. Of the comorbid emotional illnesses described in chapter 5, several pose an increased risk of suicide. ADHD is notable because one study clearly shows that depressed teenagers with this disorder choose the most lethal means to make their suicide attempt. The impulsivity associated with this disorder is what especially predisposes to an attempt. Hypomania is likewise marked by impulsivity, and when it is coupled with depression, it is usually called bipolar disorder. Doctors are just beginning to document that bipolar teens attempt suicide at twice the rate as depressed teens without hypomanic personality traits. The debate is ongoing as to whether panic disorder poses an increased risk. Until the debate gets settled, however, parents would be wise to be especially watchful of a depressed teen, especially a girl, who is prone to panic attacks.

Sexual pressure. Teenage sexuality used to be a rare indulgence in a forbidden fruit, or an occasional romantic adventure that sometimes turned into a clumsy misadventure, or a fondly remembered rite of passage saved for prom time. Not anymore. Much of the magic is gone. The dramatic change in teen sexuality has been surprisingly abrupt, occurring within the past ten years, not taking a generation or two. It has happened right under parents' noses with most of them totally unaware. How has teen sexuality changed? First, according to careful national surveys, the percentage of high school students, both male and female, who admit to having sexual intercourse is now almost 50 percent. Not too long ago it was only 20 percent. The college years were the time for high-frequency sexual behavior and experimention. The new paradigm, however, has shifted the time well into high school, and today's teens are having intercourse long before the prom. Don't think that the early teen years are safe, either. A report by the National Campaign to Prevent Teen Pregnancy found that about 20 percent of adolescents had intercourse before their fifteenth birthday. Second, teens' attitudes toward sex are much more permissive, with the majority of them considering oral sex not to be "sex" at all. Finally, sexual encounters are turning out to be more casual than planned, more sensual than romantic. They also don't necessarily lead to dating or going steady—promises are seldom given or taken. The term used for the encounters is *hooking up*. Eric told me it means whatever the couple wants it to mean—anything from kissing and groping to going all the way to "the wild thing." Often, teenagers who hook up do so randomly with whoever is convenient, and often with strangers. Sometimes the relationship lasts for several weeks or months. More often, though, it ends after several hours, not even making it until the next morning. Hooking up resumes at the next party, and not necessarily with the previous partner. It is pure mating behavior, signifying nothing more.

This new kind of high school sexual activity can be a problem unto itself by causing a fair amount of stress. After all, this culture of high-frequency, high-intensity sexual behavior spells a new requirement that teens be sexually active in order to be cool or accepted.

But the sexual activity may only be a symptom of another problem. Sex has always promised happiness, and so sexual activity can be considered a kind of medicine. This medicine has now become a legitimate prescription in high school—and even middle school for some kids. Teenagers stressed-out by overly demanding schedules, for example, may turn to this feel-good drug for a distraction or a relief. Depressed teenagers find it an especially attractive self-medication, because the acceptance that sexual partnering implies may be an antidote for the teen's feelings of isolation and worthlessness. Whether the frequent sexual activity is only a symptom or the actual problem, it is a marker of teen distress. It is no wonder, then, that mental health researchers have recently identified increased sexual activity as an important factor associated with teen suicide attempts. Add to all this the specter of STDs, or the formidable problem of an unwanted pregnancy, and it is easy to understand how teen sexuality can provide the escalation from just thinking about suicide to actually attempting it.

Emotional contagion. Eric's godmother got him a subscription to *Teen People* magazine. In November 1998, it ran a four-page story about Pierre, South Dakota, with this headline: "Eight teens from a small Midwestern town have committed suicide over the last three years. Their loved ones are determined to stop the epidemic." The story focused on Kenneth White, described his last days, and contained photographs of his tombstone and both pages of his heartrending suicide note, which his mother had laminated for safekeeping. It scared me because Eric was in the middle of his depression. I saved the article, but I never let him read it. Emotional contagion is real. It is not a statistical quirk or a fortuitous clustering of tragedies. It applies to actual suicides and to suicide attempts. The reason is that teens are immature, and they imitate other teens. Since the publication of this magazine story, researchers have nailed down one of the reasons for the contagion effect—media coverage. The more prominent the media coverage, and the longer it lasts, the greater is the contagion effect for teen suicide and suicide attempts. If we knew then what we know now, that intense story about Pierre would probably not have been written in such a sensational way, or maybe the editors would have decided not to print it at all. But media coverage is not the only way suicide news spreads. If your teen knows another teen who committed or attempted suicide, that is sufficient for contagion, and sufficient to justify a heightened alert for you. Author Andrew Solomon says the reason is that the other person's suicide makes the unthinkable now thinkable. When a member of a teen's family commits suicide, there is more than just contagion. Researchers think that multiple suicides within the same family can also be explained by a genetic effect. The statistics are frightening. If a teen's father committed suicide, the teen's risk is doubled. Or if the mother did, the teen's risk is fivefold. Studies of identical twins show the same magnitude of increased risk when one of them commits suicide.

Previous suicide attempt. Perhaps the strongest predictive factor for a completed suicide is that the teen has already attempted suicide. If this applies to your teenager, and especially if he is a boy, you ought to be on the highest possible alert, no matter how trivial or ill-conceived the first attempt seemed. "When I heard that Lauren had jumped from a second-story deck, I thought it was just some kind of kung fu stunt," her mother said. Less than two years later, Lauren took an overdose. "When he was in the tenth grade, he made a halfhearted attempt to slash his wrists," Blake's mother said. As a college sophomore, he shot himself in the head.

Step 6—If you are on heightened alert, take *immediate* action to decrease the risk of an imminent suicide attempt.

Here's what to do.

Tap into a crisis hotline. Get the phone number, give it to your teenager, and post it prominently in the house. The effectiveness of crisis hotlines is currently being studied, and the jury is not yet in. Still, teen suicide is an impulsive act, and a hotline conversation, or a recommended crisis-center visit, may use up enough time to allow the heat of the impulse to pass. Also, teen suicide is often an immature act because a teenager, poor in problem-solving and coping skills, may not know what else to do. The voice on the hotline might have enough of a solution to make a difference. In this regard, check with your son's or daughter's mental health therapist and make sure these kinds of strategies are getting taught during the therapy sessions.

Talk to your teen regularly about suicide. "After he attempted it, we talked an enormous amount," Dan's mother said. "I would ask him, 'Do you still feel suicidal? Do you want to live?' We talked a lot about all the reasons he wanted to live." There's more than just venting here, although that is important. Research has shown that talking about suicide ideation is protective. The two of you may happen onto important solutions, and your teen won't feel isolated. Even if your child seems reluctant to talk, do it anyway. Most teenagers are grateful for any intervention that will pull them back from the brink.

Keep a suicide watch. Dan attempted suicide with an overdose late at night, so his mother was especially vigilant during these vulnerable hours. "If he was in his bedroom alone, every half hour I would make up an excuse to go in. I would say something like 'You want a Coke?'" Then I would wait until he was sound asleep until I went to bed. I could tell when he was sound asleep because he really snored." She took the watch one brave and important step further. "I told everybody I knew [about his attempt]," she said. "I wanted them to help. I wanted all of them to watch." Lauren's mother could appreciate when Lauren was especially vulnerable. "The week before she would have her menstrual cycle, she would get into more of a funk. I would be around more and try to get her out of her bedroom more. 'Come do your homework downstairs in the kitchen.' Eventually, I had to be on the lookout every week. I cut back my hours at work to spend more time with her. We would just sit and watch TV or go shopping at Target. I would be there with her in the house." Eric only thought about suicide, but I kept a watch for him, too. All three of us parents will tell you it's exhausting.

Consider moving your teen back home. Researchers at the University of Texas have shown that depressed teens who feel more lonely think more about suicide. If necessary, move your teen to a college closer to home. If he is out in the workforce living on his own, suggest that he move back home. This kind of "boomerang kid" maneuver may save a life.

Try to avoid family conflicts. Of course, this is easier said than done, but at least you can cut them down to a minimum. Interpersonal conflicts, especially with parents, are known to be the most common stressors that precede a suicide attempt. This is particularly true for adolescents under the age of fifteen. "We had a fight," Dan's mother said. "It precipitated the attempt. He is a people-pleaser, especially with me. If I show any kind of disappointment, he'll follow me around the house until I'm not angry. I said, 'Enough is enough. I need my space. Go away.' He sobbed then. Nine times out of ten I give in. This time I didn't."

Watch for disruptions of interpersonal relationships. This seems to be the second most common stressor leading up to a suicide attempt, especially among older adolescents. When romantic or steady relationships with a boyfriend or girlfriend are terminated, or when serious fights with a significant person such as a coach occur, a suicide attempt may be lurking around the corner. Talk to your teen more—and intensify the watch.

After the first suicide attempt, get medical care and stay with it. Of all the authors writing about depression, Andrew Solomon pointed out an unfortunate reality: "Those who attempt tend to attempt again. No one makes much use of this fact." It is unconscionable that about 80 percent of people who attempt suicide get inadequate follow-up medical care. They get discharged from the emergency room after the overdose, and no one checks to make sure they show up for their appointment with a therapist or family doctor. Or, if they do show, most of them come for one or two visits, and that is the end of it. Adolescents are generally not compliant with psychiatric treatment. It becomes the obligation, then, of you as the parental partner to make sure the teen is inducted into treatment and stays with it as long as necessary. The night of his overdose, while Dan slept on the sofa with his head on his mother's lap, she said she was thinking, "The next day I was going to call his psychiatrist and tell him I was going to sit outside his door until he saw Dan."

7

Strategy Five
Work with Your Family Physician and Manage the Medications

Children and teenagers are not small-scale versions of adults.

Medically speaking, they are their own people. They get different kinds of pneumonia or cancer than adults. They often need their own special kinds of surgery. And sometimes they respond differently to medicines. For example, an aspirin tablet that is ordinarily safe for an adult may cause Reye's syndrome in a young child, an often fatal condition in which the liver undergoes massive and irreversible degeneration.

A worldwide debate has now sprung up as to whether children and adolescents might also respond idiosyncratically to antidepressant medications. For several years, British mental-health researchers had been observing an apparently increased incidence of suicidal thoughts and suicidal behaviors among young patients taking antidepressant medicines. The worry was that somehow the antidepressant drug itself was causing the suicidal tendencies.

The U.S. Food and Drug Administration (FDA) came to the same tentative conclusion just last September. In this country, the FDA says about 2 to 3 percent of children and teenagers taking antidepressant medication seem to manifest new suicidal thoughts or make suicide attempts. The risk seems to be greatest during the first four to six weeks after beginning the antidepressant medicine.

Does postulating a link between antidepressant medicines and suicide make good scientific sense, though?

On one hand, it would seem so. Some teens taking antidepressant medications experience anxiety, agitation, impulsiveness, panic attacks, hostility, or insomnia. When severe, these side effects could theoretically put teens at risk for worsening suicidal thoughts or behaviors. Another theory is that antidepressant drugs relieve the lethargy of depression before they relieve the hopelessness. Thus, the teen is peculiarly enlivened to put suicidal thoughts into action.

On the other hand, the conclusion seems a bit hasty. After all, suicidal thinking and suicide attempts are an intrinsic part of depression. "When suicide is part of the natural disease, then it's very hard to say that a treatment is linked to suicide," says Dr. Dianne Murphy, director of the Office of Pediatric Therapeutics at the FDA. Dr. Murphy believes that the best way to get at the truth is to study whether suicidal behavior is increased among teens who are not depressed but are taking antidepressant drugs for other reasons, such as generalized anxiety disorder or obsessive-compulsive disorder. She says that the FDA is currently considering such studies, but no launch date has yet been set.

The American College of Neuropsychopharmacology (ACN) did not come to the conclusion that antidepressant drugs could backfire. They appointed their own task force to examine the issue and found that the evidence linking these drugs to suicide was too weak to justify not using them for depression. They also pointed to the hard statistical fact that the incidence of suicide among teens has decreased as antidepressant usage has increased. Moreover, autopsies of depressed individuals show that suicide is more likely when the deceased individuals did not take the antidepressant medication that was prescribed or when they took an incorrect dose.

If your teen's doctor likewise believes that the benefits of an antidepressant drug far outweigh the risks, you must work with the doctor to manage the medication. Here are a few steps to take:

1. Be sure to tell your teen's doctor whether your teenager has ever demonstrated any suicidal tendencies.
2. After writing the initial antidepressant prescription, make sure your teen's doctor schedules the first follow-up for one week, not for one month. This is especially important because much of the suicidal thinking and behavior occurs at the onset of antidepressant therapy. Don't ever have your teen take powerful medicine without close follow-up.
3. Ask your teen's doctor if she suspects that your teen might have undiagnosed bipolar disorder. As mentioned in chapter 5, this is an extremely difficult condition to figure out in a young person. However, the mania or hypomania that is integral to the disease might get triggered or magnified by an antidepressant. The result could be disastrous. An agitated bipolar teen could find himself over-energized enough to act on a suicide impulse.
4. Periodically check the Web sites of the FDA (www.fda.gov/cder/drug/antidepressants) and the ACN (www.acnp.org/exec_summary.pdf) for the latest information on this important issue.
5. Watch for reports of new and better studies. Already, a large study of children and teens, sponsored by the National Institutes of Health and carried out without financing from drug manufacturers, was reported just last June. In that study, researchers found that teens taking antidepressant medications actually became less suicidal.

6. Finally, employ steps 1 and 2, pages 98–102, in chapter 6 to frequently assess your teen's suicide risk. A parent must keep the watch.

"It's a very confusing story out there for any parent," says Dr. David Mrazek, head of psychiatry at the Mayo Clinic. Still, he says, the risk is "very, very low" and shouldn't dissuade parents from considering an antidepressant medicine for their teen. Other adolescent psychiatrists are even more vehement. They feel that the current debate about suicide may turn out to be counterproductive by depriving many desperate teens of the very medicines that could pull them from the dark waters.

After carefully weighing the risks and benefits, your teenager's physician may suggest a course of antidepressants. This does not stigmatize your child or brand him a "crazy person." It's a logical way to treat an illness with a strong biochemical component. If you have any doubts about the validity of medication for treating depression, consider the genesis of the disease.

Stress, Brain Chemistry, and Depression

Depression is a complex disease, but it has often been regarded primarily as a stress-related disorder. Usually the stressful event that sets off depression is not of horrendous magnitude, such as an assault or a rape. That kind of event usually leads to post-traumatic stress disorder, a disease distinct from depression. Rather, the stressor is chronic and not as severe. It can be as mundane as a boy getting rejected by a girl he wants to date, or struggling to get the grades that will ensure admission to a good college.

Researchers who have created models of depression in young laboratory animals have added chronic mild stressors to the animals' environment such as disruption of the dark-light cycle, exposure to the odors of natural predators, or inescapable proximity to dominant males. You can easily extrapolate that the modern equivalents of these stressors prowl the hallways of the average American high school. Subtractions from the environment, too, such as the lack of warmth and support that occurs because of a forced separation from the mother, are equally inciting stressors. Such animals start behaving in many ways as if they were humanly depressed, and some of the depressive behavior can be reversed with antidepressant drugs such as Prozac.

Leading researchers have formulated the "kindling" hypothesis. For susceptible teenagers, they say, chronic psychosocial stress, such as unresolvable social defeat, is usually what kindles the first episode of depression. (Sometimes the bad fire never burns itself out. It smolders on, so that subsequent episodes need even less of a stressor.) What is really happening, these researchers say, is that the enormous biological apparatus in the brain and endocrine glands that responds to stress—the cells, the synapses, the chemicals, and the hormones—gets switched on and doesn't revert to a resting state, as it is supposed to, after the initial shock passes. Instead, this protective physiological machinery works overtime, and for months. And it can't properly switch itself off.

As a result, what is observable on the outside of the susceptible teenager is clinical depression. Inside, though, the stress has profoundly changed the body's biochemistry. If one probes the chemistry of the brain and the body fluids, it becomes clear that a derangement of metabolism has occurred. Scientists have intensively studied this perverse new metabolism. For example, they have routinely found elevated levels of cortisol, a stress-related hormone, in the blood, urine, saliva, and spinal fluid of depressed people. Moreover, the higher the cortisol level, the greater is the severity of the depression, and the greater is the suicide risk. When depressed people are successfully treated with antidepressant medications, their cortisol levels typically return to normal.

Studies of the neurotransmitter serotonin have also advanced our understanding of the biochemical component of depression. People with depression have been found to have lower levels of serotonin circulating in their brains. This discovery led to the development of selective serotonin reuptake inhibitors (SSRIs) such as Prozac and Zoloft, which have revolutionized the treatment of depression.

The brain is enormously complex. Many body-produced chemicals other than cortisol and serotonin play a role in clinical depression. Other substances such as norepinephrine, dopamine, thyroid hormone, and obscure neurotransmitters with barely pronounceable names are receiving equally intense laboratory scrutiny. But you don't have to become an expert in brain chemistry to be an effective parental partner. You simply have to understand that depression involves a biochemical cascade of changes, and medication is an important tool for putting it right.

The brain has a marvelous plasticity, and changes in body biochemistry may cause the brain to rewire itself. This can work to a person's advantage. For example, scientists have performed elegant experiments with blind people learning to read braille. The portion of their brain responsible for finger sensations enlarges with beneficial new circuits dedicated for this purpose. However, when emotional illnesses such as depression rewire the brain, the brain develops new pathological neural circuits, built by cortisol or some other chemical messenger, that give rise to torturous or self-destructive emotions. Scientists are now using sophisticated brain-scan technologies to detect these new circuits, even aiming to diagnose depression or other mental illnesses based on the scan results alone. The mind is the sum of the brain's circuits. That is why pharmacologists, searching for new drugs for depression, aim to dampen these pathological new circuits or activate compensatory good ones.

Choosing an Antidepressant Rationally

The overwhelming evidence that depression largely represents a derangement of brain biochemistry justifies the use of an antidepressant drug as first-line therapy for your depressed teenager. Your family doctor has two chief concerns when writing the prescription for your teen. The first is to get an improvement in symptoms as quickly as possible and improve your child's functioning. The second is to be sure the prescribed drug has an excellent safety profile with the fewest possible side effects. In this regard, the initial prescription most likely will be for a drug from the class of antidepressants called SSRIs.

You may encounter some initial resistance from your teenager. Some young people will feel embarrassed. Some will feel stigmatized. But almost all desperately want help. In fact, most are relieved when they get a prescription and hear an explanation of how it works, often saying something like "You mean I don't have to feel this way?"

As a partner with your teen's health-care providers, you can make a crucial difference when it comes time to write that initial prescription and possibly subsequent prescriptions for other drugs. You can make your doctor's process more sophisticated than just trial and error, which is how it was for Lauren. "She had been on a bazillion drugs," her mother said. "They weren't working for her. The doctor added drugs. He changed drugs. He increased the dose. It took three years to find the right ones."

You may not realize it, but you have immensely valuable information that can do a lot to help refine the doctor's choice of which antidepressant to use. The choice is crucial for efficacy and for your teen's acceptance of the drug. Here are six subjects you ought to discuss with your teen's physician before the prescription gets written:

1. Comorbidity. If you think your teenager has generalized anxiety disorder or ADHD, he is already agitated. It makes no sense, then, for your doctor to prescribe antidepressants that cause agitation as a side effect. Especially effective drugs that cause a minimum of "activation" symptoms such as anxiety, tremors, and restlessness are Luvox and Celexa. Also, tell your physician if you suspect your teen has an eating disorder. Wellbutrin was developed to be especially free of side effects, but the electrolyte imbalances of young people with eating disorders predispose them to seizures when they take this drug.

2. Fatigue. Some depressed teenagers mope a lot and sleep too much. "She would sleep all day in the fetal position," Lauren's mother said. Tell your doctor if your teen is fatigued or tired much of the time, because antidepressants such as Prozac and Zoloft are especially good at "energizing" them.

3. Insomnia. The previously mentioned drugs that have sedating side effects, Luvox and Celexa, are especially appropriate here. Your doctor can exploit this side effect for your insomniac teen's advantage.

4. Concern about weight gain. Only a few commonly used antidepressants have this side effect, but you certainly want to avoid these drugs if your teenager would be especially prone to discontinue taking the drug because of some extra pounds.

5. Herbal supplements. Teens may ignore telling their doctor they are using herbal or nutritional supplements, assuming the supplements are not "drugs." This is simply not true, and some of these substances are quite powerful. Saint-John's-wort, technically known as hypericum, causes some of the same side effects as the SSRIs, namely, frequent urination or sexual dysfunction. If the doctor prescribes an SSRI antidepressant for a teenager who is also taking Saint-John's-wort, the combined side effects might become burdensome. Moreover, this substance is capable of adverse interactions with other prescription drugs. (For example, it interferes with some drugs for cancer and AIDS, and it has clearly been implicated in the rejection of two transplanted hearts.) Don't let your teen self-medicate with herbal remedies. Natural does not necessarily mean benign.

6. *Which antidepressant worked well for other members of your family.* One logical factor in choosing a drug would be to favor the drug that worked for you, your spouse, or your other children. "Lauren's [final] doctor was right on," her mother said. "He wanted to know what [antidepressants] I tried and what worked for me." His question was based on the supposition that for some people depression may be genetic. In other words, if the susceptibility to the disease is carried on a gene, then, too, so could the depression's responsiveness to certain medications. Thus, both susceptibility and responsiveness may be transmitted to the next generation as a DNA package deal. Scientific studies indicate that a good response to Fluvox may be anticipated if a depressed first-degree relative responded well. More studies are needed to pinpoint how much of a determinant this "familial factor" will turn out to be.

Measuring the Response to the Initial Treatment

The goal of initial treatment with the antidepressant medicine is to get a prompt beneficial response, that is, a significant and measurable improvement in your teenager's depressive symptoms. How do you know if it's working? It's up to you as the parental partner to closely monitor your teen's depressive symptoms. After all, you know your teen best. Your doctor will appreciate your partnering efforts, because your assessment is firsthand, straight from the trenches. As Dan's mother so aptly said, "You know what? I live with this every day. I know what's going on."

One way to achieve a sensible measurement of improvement is by comparing the scores from a symptom rating chart your teen fills out just before starting the antidepressant medicine with the one filled out several weeks later when returning to the doctor's office for the first follow-up visit. In this manner, you and the doctor will have an objective appraisal of whether your teen is on the right course. If not, an adjustment or change of medication is in order.

Just before starting the antidepressant drug, ask your teenager to complete the symptom chart below. Have her circle the appropriate rating number for each item. Then total the score and record it. Make sure you examine your teen's ratings to see if they jibe with your impressions and write your notes on the chart as well.

Symptom Chart—Before Starting Treatment

	Seldom or never	Some of the time	Much of the time	Almost always
1. I feel sad, blue, or down in the dumps.	0	1	2	3
2. I am angry or irritable.	0	1	2	3
3. I can't get to sleep right away, or I sleep too much.	0	1	2	3
4. My appetite and weight are changing.	0	1	2	3
5. I get tired a lot and can't figure out why.	0	1	2	3
6. It is hard to concentrate.	0	1	2	3
7. I feel anxious or hyper.	0	1	2	3
8. I am pessimistic about the future.	0	1	2	3
9. I don't enjoy the things I used to do.	0	1	2	3
10. I no longer pursue the things that used to interest me.	0	1	2	3
11. I think my family and friends don't need me.	0	1	2	3
12. I think about killing myself.	0	1	2	3

Total Score _____

This same symptom chart is printed below. Have your teen fill it out the day of the first return appointment and total the score. Again, make sure the ratings jibe with your observations and jot down your notes. Give copies of both completed charts to your family doctor. This kind of a rating chart should provide a fairly good idea of what degree of response your teen is achieving with the medication. Otherwise, the doctor would have to rely on often imprecise statements from the teen like "The world seems better" or "I don't feel so bad anymore." Teenage boys in particular may make remarkably inexact statements because they have more difficulty talking about emotional issues than do teenage girls.

Symptom Chart—After Starting Treatment

	Seldom or never	Some of the time	Much of the time	Almost always
1. I feel sad, blue, or down in the dumps.	0	1	2	3
2. I am angry or irritable.	0	1	2	3
3. I can't get to sleep right away, or I sleep too much.	0	1	2	3
4. My appetite and weight are changing.	0	1	2	3
5. I get tired a lot and can't figure out why.	0	1	2	3
6. It is hard to concentrate.	0	1	2	3
7. I feel anxious or hyper.	0	1	2	3
8. I am pessimistic about the future.	0	1	2	3
9. I don't enjoy the things I used to do.	0	1	2	3
10. I no longer pursue the things that used to interest me.	0	1	2	3
11. I think my family and friends don't need me.	0	1	2	3
12. I think about killing myself.	0	1	2	3

Total Score _____

Researchers are trying to figure out how much of a change in the score on a symptom rating chart constitutes a minimally acceptable improvement. There are almost as many different opinions as there are charts and researchers. Nevertheless, the sum total of their opinions indicates that there should be about a 50 percent improvement in the ratings of the depressive symptoms. That is, your teen's score on the follow-up-visit chart ought to be half or less of the score on the pretreatment chart. Still, depression is a complex illness that can't entirely be expressed as a mere score. Make sure you ask for the doctor's interpretation of the charts and of any notes you made on them.

Despite a seemingly robust response to the antidepressant medication, in the case of at least one-third of depressed teens, the score may not drop much below 50 percent. In other words, these teens are left with residual symptoms, the most common ones being anhedonia, fatigue, or a sleep disturbance. Don't settle for this. The residual symptoms are a flashing warning light. They signify danger for both a high rate of relapse of the current depressive episode, and a high rate of recurrence of future episodes.

Residual symptoms have several possible explanations. Discuss all these possibilities with your teen's doctor. In this way, the doctor will get a better idea of how to proceed to achieve an even better response.

One explanation is that treatment with the initial SSRI has not yet been optimized. A landmark study done a decade ago showed that only 11 percent of primary care physicians wrote antidepressant prescriptions that were optimal for dose and length of treatment. SSRIs typically take four to six weeks to kick in, although some people feel a difference in two weeks. Sometimes twelve weeks must pass before an optimal response is observed. Dosage is another consideration—one size does not fit all. Ask the prescribing doctor whether the dose of the current antidepressant needs to be increased.

If the doctor thinks your teen has taken the drug in the right dose for the right length of time, but your teen's symptoms have not significantly improved, he will likely consider switching to another SSRI. After one SSRI failure, however, the response rate for the second SSRI is only 50 percent. Watch for side effects if a second SSRI is started. Sometimes, the second choice was not the first choice because of its worse side-effect profile.

If switching to a second SSRI is not an option or has already failed, adding a second medication that is not itself an antidepressant, such as buspirone or lithium, may augment the action of the SSRI. If lithium is chosen, make sure you quiz the doctor about its necessity. Lithium can be an effective drug against depression, but it requires periodic monitoring by venipuncture or fingerstick of its level in your teen's blood to accurately control the dosage. In addition, thyroid function and kidney function need watching.

Switching to an altogether different class of antidepressants such as the TCAs (tricyclic antidepressants) may be in order as a last-ditch stand, but these "other class" drugs, on average, don't work as well for young people as for adults, or they have the potential for worrisome side effects. Ask your doctor if all other options have indeed been exhausted before turning to the tricyclics.

Are you or your spouse currently depressed? Mood disorders aggregate in families. Studies show that one-third to one-half of depressed teenagers have parents who have a mood disorder at the same time. Successful treatment of a parent's concurrent depression speeds the teen's recovery from her own depression. Tell the doctor if your own depression is going untreated. This could be slowing your teen's improvement, and the doctor may wrongly ascribe responsibility to the drug. The result could be an inappropriate escalation of the drug's dose, with a risk of more side effects for your teen, or a switch to another drug that may have less of a safety profile. The correct approach in these circumstances is to get your own depression promptly treated.

The residual symptoms might also be signs of a different problem. They may represent dysfunctional personality traits, such as deficient social skills, that actually antedated the depressive episode and made your teen vulnerable to depression's inciting events. Or the residual symptoms may represent new personality traits that postdate the onset of the depressive episode and are resulting psychological "scars." In either case, medications alone won't be the complete answer. As a parent, you know your teen best. If you believe either of these alternatives may be true, this is another time to be a proactive partner and push your doctor for a referral to a mental health therapist. Don't let up until the referral gets made.

The Ultimate Goal Is Remission

You want more than a response to medication—you want a remission. You want your teen's suffering to end. You want your teenager back on track, healthy and hopeful, with self-worth growing, and free of suicidal thoughts. Teenagers who do not achieve a remission on drugs will likely demonstrate prolonged problems with poor social skills, dysfunctional attitudes, and impaired problem-solving abilities. Moreover, if some of the major depressive symptoms fail to abate, the chances for a recurrence of a major depressive episode within five years remain high. Finally, continuation of only a few of the major symptoms may morph into dysthymia, a torturous and debilitating condition of continuous grinding mild depression that lasts a lifetime.

While your teen is being treated with drugs, have her fill out the symptom rating chart every month or so. A score of about six or more ought to be a warning. It indicates a remission has not yet been achieved. No remission is your signal to push especially hard for a referral to a mental health therapist—and for more than just two or three visits. Research evidence is now accumulating that the best chance for a remission in an adolescent occurs with the combination of medications and psychotherapy. Advocating for your teen now may save her a lifetime of misery. It may save her a psychiatric hospitalization. It may save her life.

However, your family doctor may need evidence for the health insurer to justify a referral to a mental health therapist. In fact, the evidence is now being written in the accumulating scientific studies that show that teens who do not achieve remission will cost the insurer more money in the long run. These teens make more ER visits, require more frequent hospitalizations, attempt suicide more often, and suffer more relapses and recurrences. All of these unfortunate outcomes are expensive in the long run for the health insurer. If necessary, ask your doctor to look up the studies.

Continuation Treatment for the First Episode

Once your son or daughter has achieved an acceptable response on antidepressant medications, how long should the drug be continued? The purpose of continuation treatment is to prevent a relapse of the current depressive episode. Most professionals recommend that a teen continue taking the antidepressant medication for about six months after the symptoms of the first episode have abated, and more likely for nine months. Sadly, studies reveal that only half of depressed patients actually receive this minimum recommended therapy. This is where the parent-partner makes a difference. Remind your doctor that one of the biggest mistakes made with antidepressants is to stop them too soon. Don't worry about long-term side effects of long-term therapy. Over the past fifteen years, literally millions of prescriptions for SSRIs have been written. These drugs have proved to be remarkably free of adverse effects on the function of any organ or physiological system. They are so lacking in side effects that many nondepressed people opt to take SSRIs to enhance their mood and functioning.

Maintenance Treatment to Prevent Future Episodes

No one really knows yet how long to treat after the first episode is resolved in order to prevent a second episode. This is a highly controversial area in contemporary psychiatry, and there are no firm answers about this kind of maintenance treatment. Since teenage depression is a more serious form of the disease, the chance of a recurrence is high—50 percent. Still, this means 50 percent of teens will not have a recurrence. If your teen has received at least six to nine months of continuation treatment for the first episode, and it has resolved well, an appropriate choice seems to be no further drug treatment. It would seem wise simply to wait and watch. Watch diligently, though. Eric received adequate treatment for his first episode, but he experienced a second, although milder, episode during his sophomore year in college. Your doctor will have to carefully individualize and weigh all aspects of your teen's depression, particularly if the first episode was especially rocky. I still look back and wonder whether Eric should have been prescribed some maintenance treatment.

What if your teen has already had two episodes and the aim is to prevent a third? Because two episodes during one's youth signifies a particularly malevolent form of depression, some professional organizations feel compelled to take a stand on how long to treat after the second episode resolves. The World Health Organization has recommended two years of maintenance treatment for people who have suffered two episodes of serious depression. This is pretty much the thinking of U.S. psychiatrists also, with a few saying that three years might be better. So, if your teenager is now being treated for a serious second episode, ask your doctor to consider prescribing maintenance antidepressants for at least two years. The British Association for Psychopharmacology has gone further and recommends that people who have suffered two episodes of severe depression should take the drugs indefinitely. To repeat, the biggest mistake made with antidepressants is to stop them too soon.

These professional recommendations have been conscientiously weighed, but they need to be tested by more research studies with teenagers. What should be done until the studies get done? The insight, intuition, and common sense of parents are valuable substitutes for research data to judge whether a particular teen should take antidepressants continuously for several years. Although there might be slight risks to taking antidepressants for a prolonged time, consider that the risks of not taking them might be enormous. "I think the success was because of me," Dan's mother said. "I kept pushing. I made appointments when he needed more medication or when the medication wasn't right. Things finally stabilized for him." To come to a sensible conclusion about maintenance treatment for your teen, you should bring up these issues with the doctor:

- The severity of your teen's recent depressive episode
- The difficulty in getting a significant response or a remission
- Whether you or any other of the teen's close relatives have been depressed
- Whether your teen lacks insight into any cognitive factors that led up to the depression
- Whether an ongoing family dysfunction will not promptly be solved

- Whether your teen has any chronic predisposing factors that cannot be resolved well, such as ADHD, a chronic illness, or a physical impairment
- A previous suicide attempt

If you and your doctor conclude that prophylactic maintenance treatment for several years seems advisable, the recommended dose ought to be the original dose used for the acute episode, not a diminished dose. Remember that the unfortunate consequence of undertreatment is recurrence of another depressive episode.

Noncompliance—When Teenagers Won't Take Their Medicine

Antidepressant drugs won't work if your son or daughter won't take them. On their own, young people may discontinue taking the medicine. On average, they do this after about ten weeks of therapy. The reason they give most commonly is that they are "feeling better" and no longer need the drug. Beware—fully one-fourth of them will not tell you or their doctor. As a parental partner you'll have to check on compliance periodically throughout the treatment.

Side effects are the second most common reason for noncompliance. The side effects of antidepressants are mild in comparison to those caused by many other kinds of drugs. The problem, though, is that antidepressants must be taken for prolonged periods, and so the duration of the side effects becomes especially bothersome.

In particular, teens complain about two side effects.

One is sexual dysfunction. With the SSRI class of drugs, both sexes experience diminished libido. "He said he had no sexual urges at all," Dan's mother said. "He said he felt like an 'it.'" In addition, girls complain of attenuated orgasm or absent orgasm. Boys notice erectile dysfunction, delayed ejaculation, or painful ejaculation. Some teenagers worry that the sexual dysfunction may be permanent or represent something serious. They might even be worried enough to consult gynecologists or urologists, sometimes without their parents' knowledge.

You may not like it, but with teen sexuality sharply on the rise, this may be an important consideration, especially for college students. "One of my friends who was taking an antidepressant logged on to one of those drugstore Web sites to get Viagra," Eric told me during his first year at college. "You tell them a bunch of lies, like you had a physical done and all the papers are at your doctor's office, and the Web site doctor will mail you the prescription."

Doctors call this technique of treating drug side effects with other drugs "polypharmacy." When young people do it on their own, it can develop into a dangerous habit. If sexual side effects are a serious and valid issue for your older teenager, consider speaking to the doctor about switching to a medication that is better at preserving sexual function, such as Wellbutrin or Remeron. You may disapprove, but still find it preferable to having him fool around with Viagra or even cocaine to stimulate sexuality.

The other particularly troublesome side effect is weight gain. Much to our chagrin, body image is an obsession with many adolescent girls, and it is now becoming more important among boys. This side effect often occurs insidiously. At first, there may be a mild weight loss, because of side effects of decreased appetite or nausea. These wear off after several weeks, and then the pounds may start to accumulate. Weight gain might be a deal-breaker for your teenager. If so, Wellbutrin or Serzone are alternative choices to minimize or even avoid this problem.

The kinds of antidepressants your doctor will prescribe are not addictive, and cessation of the drug will not cause a withdrawal syndrome. But if your teenager stops taking the drug, she may still come down with a "discontinuation" syndrome. The symptoms are predominantly physical, not psychological, and may include dizziness, numbness, headache, tremors, nightmares, nausea, and anxiety. About one-third of teenagers who discontinue their medicines will experience this kind of syndrome. It is mild, not dangerous, and lasts only several days or weeks. The real danger, though, is that you or your doctor may interpret the undetected noncompliance as a worsening of the depression. If the erroneous conclusion is made that the current treatment is ineffective, your teen could needlessly be switched to a different drug with less of a safety profile.

When the appropriate time comes to stop the drug, a discontinuation syndrome is a definite consideration. Don't misinterpret it as a relapse or recurrence of the depression. Tapering the drug, rather than stopping it abruptly, avoids the syndrome.

Some teenagers will refuse to take any antidepressant. They worry that medications will inhibit their creativity, dull their intelligence, or detract from their individuality. "She told me she valued her own brain chemistry," Chloe's mother said. "She said, 'If I took happy pills, the happiness would be artificial, and I might get to like the artificial happiness better than my natural happiness.' She said she valued her emotions, and there might be a reason for them. She thought the depression was an evolutionary segment in her life."

If your teenager refuses any prescription from the doctor, make sure you read chapter 11 on adjunctive treatments. For mild depression, brisk exercise almost every day can prove to be as effective as antidepressants.

Treatment-Resistant Depression

One-third of teenagers won't get much benefit from antidepressants. They will get a meager response or no response at all. This is a calamity, because depression is a serious and even life-threatening illness. Don't assume that the prescribing doctor will have time to do the detective work. You'll need to assume some responsibility for making sure this is indeed treatment-resistant depression. Many cases will turn out to be something other than depression. Here is a list of alternative explanations:

- Noncompliance is a frequent cause of spurious treatment failure. Diligently quiz your teenager about whether she has taken her medication and how regularly.
- Treatment may not yet have been optimized. Review with the doctor whether all reasonable drug substitutions and additions have been tried. If the doctor seems uncertain, consult another doctor.
- A frequent possibility is that a teenager is continuing to abuse drugs or alcohol. In this situation, some of the depressive symptoms improve, but the ongoing addiction makes other symptoms persist.
- Another possibility is that your teenager actually is dysthymic. The acute episode of major depression may have resolved, but the symptoms of the simmering dysthymia continue to show themselves, masquerading as a treatment failure.
- The treatment failure may not be of the depression but of a comorbid condition, such as bipolar disorder, ADHD, or anxiety disorder.
- An unaddressed or continuing family dysfunction may be particularly contributory, such as abuse or parental addiction.

If none of these considerations apply, and the treatment failure appears to be correctly that, what can you do?

When optimal drug therapy and psychotherapy fail, and when the teenager is trapped in the depths of oppressive depression, electroconvulsive therapy (ECT) is a legitimate consideration. Unfortunately, ECT has been stigmatized by a history of indiscriminate overuse, by melodramatic movies, and by unfounded claims of enfeebling side effects.

Strident antipsychiatry groups are trying to perpetuate the stigma. They are just as unenlightened as those who stigmatize depression as a character flaw rather than a treatable disease. It's time to ignore the rhetoric and clip any resistance you might have to the idea.

Yes, most parents who have given consent for their children and teenagers to receive ECT found the prospect frightening. However, consider this. Modern ECT appears to be the quickest, safest, and most effective form of treatment for severe depression and severe bipolar disorder. Up to 90 percent of people respond, and seemingly miraculous benefits show themselves in as little as five days from starting the treatments. Dick Cavett began experiencing incapacitating episodes of depression as a college student. Eventually, he had no option but to try ECT. "Look who's back among the living," he is quoted as saying. "It was like a magic wand." Modern ECT may also be a lifesaver, for example, for a teenager who is in imminent danger of suicide, and who should not be allowed to wait three or four weeks to get an uncertain benefit from antidepressant drugs. The American Psychiatric Association has published an information pamphlet about ECT on its Web site, and you can log on at www.psych.org/public_info/ECT. Even today, some mental health professionals hold on to the stigma attached to ECT, but when nothing else has worked for your teenager, and when she is nonfunctional, continually harms herself, or is contemplating suicide, it's your duty to broach the issue with the doctor or therapist.

Antianxiety Agents

Anxiety accompanies almost every emotional illness, and it is especially common with depression. Sometimes it is a symptom. Sometimes it is a full-blown diagnosable anxiety disorder. Anxiety is typified by the fight-or-flight response: the heart races, breathing quickens, the skin sweats, and a feeling of jumpiness and apprehension comes over the person. Add these uncomfortable sensations to the agony of depression and you can see how your teen winds up in an emotional firestorm. Sometimes the anxiety eases with the SSRI antidepressant. However, when it doesn't, your doctor may add an antianxiety drug, a tranquilizer, to ease your teen's agitation. These drugs will also help an insomniac teen get some sleep. Often the drug is of the benzodiazepine (BZD) class, and you probably know some of the names: Valium, Xanax, Serax, or Klonopin. As a parent-partner, you have a number of important concerns when your teen gets a BZD prescription.

Fatigue. Tiredness and daytime sleepiness are the most common side effects. If your depressed teen is already withdrawn or lethargic, this picture may worsen as she becomes calmer. Your doctor needs to know about the worsening somnolence.

Athletic activities. Muscle weakness is a common side effect. Some teens will lose a bit of coordination and manual dexterity. Some will even have slurred speech. Although he may complain of worsened athletic performance, these effects usually disappear after several weeks. Conversely, some teens say the disappearance of the anxiety improved their performance.

School performance. An underestimated side effect of the BZDs is the impairment they may cause for cognitive tasks. Moreover, many teens are unaware that their cognitive abilities are being compromised by the medication. You probably want to check with your teen's teachers to see if school performance is deteriorating. If so, make the teachers aware of the reason, especially if your child is also experiencing the side effect of fatigue.

Driving. BZDs impair alertness and concentration. It's no wonder, then, that several studies have documented that drivers taking these drugs are at increased risk for serious automobile accidents.

Drinking. For some people who take mild BZDs, alcohol is additive. In other words, after one BZD pill, the first drink acts like the second. But for others, the effect is synergistic—the first drink is like the fourth. You must warn your teen about the risks involved in driving and engaging in hazardous activities and sports, and be especially alert to alcohol consumption. Eric needed to take benzodiazepines for a while, and during that time I told him that I was his "permanent designated driver." If he thought he was impaired by alcohol, fatigue, or something else, he could call me for a ride, twenty-four hours a day, seven days a week, no questions asked.

Reappearance of anxiety. Your teen may have periods when the anxiety that was previously controlled seems mysteriously to reappear. Often this means the teen has stopped taking the drug because he was starting to feel better or didn't like the side effects. The error here is to increase the dose of the BZD when a resumption is merely all that is necessary.

Withdrawal. Unless your teen has been using BZDs daily for more than about four months, stopping the medication should not result in a withdrawal syndrome. The longer the BZD is taken, though, the greater is the likelihood your teen will experience a withdrawal syndrome, especially if the drug is not tapered slowly. If the drug has been used for longer than eight months, the chances of a withdrawal syndrome are fifty-fifty. Sweating, dizziness, headaches, restlessness, tremulousness, hyperventilation, and even an increased sensitivity to sound are typical symptoms. They last a few days to a few weeks.

Overdose. Fatalities are rare with pure BZD overdose. Recovery even from a coma caused by a BZD overdose is rapid and seldom results in any serious long-term consequences. However, when combined with alcohol, narcotics, barbiturates, or antidepressants of the TCA class, the danger increases greatly. Breathing may stop, or blood pressure may collapse. The outcome may be fatal.

Switching medications. Buspirone is an antianxiety agent with no sedative side effects, no interaction with alcohol, and no potential for abuse. If your teen experiences too many BZD side effects, ask your doctor about a switch to buspirone. More important, if an antianxiety drug will be needed continuously for many months, buspirone is likely preferable to a potentially addictive BZD. Its major disadvantage is that the relief of anxiety is slow—taking one to two weeks—whereas the BZDs will bring relief in several hours. The prompt relief typical of BZDs is important for those teens who show some impulsivity. They may not have the self-control to wait out the anxiety while the buspirone is gradually taking effect.

Trading medications. A survey done in 2003 by the Centers for Disease Control and Prevention showed that 10 percent of teenagers will share prescribed medicines with other teens. The most common ones are acne medicines such as Acutane, but psychoactive drugs are a close second on the list. Eric told me it is common among college students to "borrow" a tranquilizer from another student. If the drug is a powerful BZD, and if it gets ingested with alcohol, the possible synergistic effect may result in a seriously impaired driver. A particular hazard around the dormitory, Eric tells me, is that students often leave their prescription bottles out in plain sight. "I can tell you what someone's medical problems are just by walking into their room," he said. With such ready accessibility, a lot of borrowing gets done without the lender's permission. Worse yet, a pill bottle out in the open is an invitation to an overdose for those depressed teens who see no other way out of the darkness.

8

Strategy Six
Find the Right Therapist

She was twenty-four and deathly afraid of spiders. She was answering the advertisement in the Montreal newspaper asking for research volunteers with phobias. A team of doctors at that city's Notre Dame Hospital were trying to get a bit of an answer to the biggest and most pressing question in psychiatry in this decade—does successful talk therapy, without any use of psychoactive medicines, change the brain's chemicals and neural circuits? The leader of the team, Dr. Mario Beauregard, specifically wanted to scan this volunteer's head to see if successful talk therapy to make her unafraid of spiders could rewire her brain.

Dr. Beauregard enrolled her in a twelve-hour program of cognitive-behavioral therapy. She heard lectures about how beneficial spiders are and was coaxed and coached to peer into containers of living spiders. She diligently completed the assigned homework, touching color photographs of spiders, and finished the therapy with honors. Now, she could even pet a tarantula. It was time for the scan, something called a functional MRI. Dr. Beauregard was going to compare this one to her pretreatment scan obtained just prior to the talk therapy.

He found the results exciting enough to publish in a prominent medical journal. Before the cognitive behavioral therapy, two areas of her brain responsible for fear and for catastrophic thinking always switched themselves on when she viewed a videotape of moving spiders. After the therapy, however, the scan showed these areas were deactivated. The switches in her brain had been rewired, and the neural circuits for spider fear were thus rendered obsolete. Dr Beauregard couldn't escape the obvious conclusion: "Change the mind and you change the brain."

The science of imaging the brain to detect changes in its neural circuitry after successful talk therapy is in its infancy. It's been only about a decade since scientists first discovered that psychotherapy could change the blood flow and the metabolism of critical parts of the brain in people with obsessive-compulsive disorder. In the last several years there have been hints that the same is true for depression. English scientists have performed brain scans on depressed people who underwent successful interpersonal therapy, a proven kind of psychotherapy that helps the depressed person understand the low mood in terms of role disputes or interpersonal deficits. Then, the therapist teaches the depressed person new strategies to resolve the disputes and improve social skills. With a technically sophisticated form of scanning called single photon-emission computed tomography, these scientists showed that the therapy was normalizing the brain metabolism of the depressed people. Blood was now flowing throughout their brains in a pattern nearly identical to that of someone who had never been depressed. American scientists in Los Angeles replicated these results with positron-emission tomography. Owing to the development of these sophisticated research tools, the evidence is beginning to accumulate. Talk therapy for depression changes the biology of the brain.

It's fashionable nowadays to proclaim, "Freud is dead." The scans prove this isn't quite true. Actually, Freud was not a fraud, he was just wrong a lot, and many of his theories applied only to neurotic Viennese citizens of the nineteenth century. The real calamity is that other schools of psychiatry and psychology have been dragged down along with him, unjustifiably so. Personally, I am delighted the scans are quashing the wags who bash any kind of talk therapy. Their criticism is ill-founded, because they ignore that the mind is unbelievably complex, and our understanding of it, even today, is rather tenuous.

Antidepressant drugs are not the magic bullet against the demon. Research studies do not show antidepressant drugs to be uniformly more effective than psychotherapy. The effect of the drugs wears off almost as soon as they are stopped, whereas psychotherapy can show an enduring effect for months or years. Finally, evidence is emerging that psychotherapy can prevent the onset of the first episode of depression in people who are susceptible. If we believe that drugs alone can be the best answer to complex behavioral problems, we should expect the development of a pill for a troubled marriage or deficient parenting skills, but it doesn't seem possible.

The biological workings of our brain's synapses and neurotransmitters go a long way to explain our emotions, but only in part. The workings of the psychological mind still present a logical and compelling framework for questioning why we do the things we do, and why we might feel that we are worthless and life is hopeless. The answers to depression lie not on one branch of the dichotomy, biology or psychology. Rather, the scans prove that biology and psychology intertwine. Like the brain it assaults, depression is so complex that it defies being reduced to a simple formula or a single explanation.

While biologists are making great strides to explain depression, psychologists are showing that the dimensions of the personality play a crucial role, especially in the early-onset and recurrent type of depression that affects teenagers. This was best demonstrated by a study that showed that certain personality traits could predict the outcome of treatment nearly twenty years afterward. Specifically, the more "neurotic" the personality was at the onset of the depression, the less likely there would be a good recovery from the depression years later. In other words, excess fears, insecurities, and illogical thoughts worked their frightful mischief for decades, and despite any biological treatment. Perhaps it is no wonder, then, that Andrew Solomon wrote, "A sense of humor might be the best indicator you will recover." There's more to it than humor, of course. Resilience, self-knowledge, perspective, and faith are other qualities that foster recovery. But it's clear that temperament and personality make a substantial difference.

The Power of Combined Therapy

Drug therapy and psychotherapy are both powerful weapons against a depressive episode. Curiously, the two modalities are often viewed as being in competition with each other. This is not the case, because each has distinct advantages. Wouldn't it seem sensible then to combine the two modalities to achieve a more robust treatment? The practice guidelines that most doctors follow, in fact, do recommend this when the episode is severe. Studies of these kinds of depressed patients best demonstrate the power of psychotherapy and the particular benefits of combined treatment.

For example, one typical study has shown that combined therapy can do a better job in preventing a relapse of the current depressive episode than can antidepressant drug therapy alone. Even with modern antidepressants, and in adequate dosages, residual symptoms are common, and residual symptoms have scientifically been proved to be dreaded heralds for a relapse. However, when patients with these symptoms get prompt referrals for psychotherapy and take their medication, too, the relapse rate can be cut in half. This kind of protection from a relapse can go on for as long as two years.

Even more impressive is that combined psychotherapy seems effective in preventing a second episode. It is as if the psychotherapy reduces the vulnerability to depression. This should be no surprise since the aim of many kinds of psychotherapy is to give the person a new talent—the ability to inspect and correct one's thoughts. Thus, negative biases are rejected, and dysfunctional or pessimistic attitudes are cast aside. A few critics will disparage these studies, saying that some of these depressed people may actually be experiencing unrecorded recurrences; that is, they don't come to their doctors for treatment because they are treating themselves. After all, in their psychotherapy they learned new coping skills and new problem-solving skills. This is the kind of criticism I enjoy hearing. Even if the recurrence rate were somewhat higher than we think, this kind of insightful self-treating individual, even though perhaps depressed again, is still much better off than one who is powerless against the disease, having learned no new skills from a wisdomless pill. As I've watched Eric over these four years since his first episode, I see occasional bits of evidence that the depression might recur. Each time I shudder. Yet, Eric will often reply to my inquiries with reassuring answers like "I'm better off now" or "I understand so much more now, I can't believe I thought high school was so bad." I think he knows when trouble is brewing—and how to stay out of it.

The statistics for recurrence are frightening. For newly depressed teenagers, the chances of a second episode are 50 percent. For teenagers with a second episode, the chances for a third are 80 percent. And the chances then for a fourth are an astonishing 90 percent. These statistics ought to command our attention. With the recurrence rate so high, everything possible ought to be done to protect against repeated depression.

The final justification for combined therapy comes from common sense. Because of their bothersome side effects, you would expect that the noncompliance rate for teenagers taking antidepressants would be high. Scientific studies confirm this suspicion. The noncompliance rate can be as high as 44 percent for patients taking antidepressants, with 20 percent being noncompliant after only one month of treatment, and 40 percent after three months. Psychotherapy is a hedge against potentially dangerous noncompliance.

Does Your Teenager Need Psychotherapy?

Doctors admit they haven't researched this question often enough. So far, though, they have come up with one solid recommendation. A depressed person, they say, needs a psychotherapist whenever the depressive episode seems severe. They define severe according to that person's score on a rating scale of depressive symptoms. Ask your teen's doctor to do this kind of psychometric evaluation with the standardized tests commercially available. Or give him a copy of the symptom rating chart from chapter 7 that your teen filled out. Share your opinions, but, like a good partner, ask for the doctor's interpretation, too. Anytime your teen's symptoms could be scored as severe, whether it's at the beginning of antidepressant treatment or several months into it, ask your doctor about the advisability of combined therapy.

There are other reasons a psychotherapist seems necessary. Some of these are hints from scientific studies; others are pure parental common sense.

Previous suicide attempt, or strong suicide ideation. Talk therapy in such instances is mandatory.

A comorbid emotional illness. The incidence of a second emotional illness heaped on top of teen depression is about 50 percent. The incidence of a third emotional illness is about 15 percent. To assume that medications can address the large number of issues stemming from multiple emotional illnesses is to believe that modern drugs are indeed panaceas.

A comorbid medical illness. For adults, higher rates of depression, and poorer outcomes, accompany medical illnesses such as diabetes, stroke, or chronic heart disease. Worse yet, these people do not experience increased rates of treatment for their depression. This means they are underserved. Make sure your teen is not underserved. Asthma, migraine headaches, diabetes, epilepsy, hearing impairment, or inflammatory bowel disease are relatively common during the teen years. If they seem in any way debilitating, or if they interfere with the maturational tasks of adolescence, ask your doctor about the advisability of combined therapy.

Noncompliance with antidepressant medications. A mental health therapist can fill in the gaps left when the pills aren't taken. "Michelle would flush her pills down the toilet," her father said. You have to do some detective work to determine if your teenager is taking the medication regularly.

"Depressogenic" habits or thinking that antedated the depressive episode. Certain unhealthy personality characteristics have been implicated in the etiology of depression. Psychologists often point to the "negative triad": the teenager is negative about herself, her future, and her world. This kind of "stinky thinking," they say, might actually predispose a susceptible teen to depression. Medicines can't usually correct the distorted thinking, but talk therapy

may. Other traits and habits that may lay the foundation for depression include interpersonal dependency, relentless self-criticism, pessimism, and perfectionism in the face of unmet personal goals. Only you will know whether your teen possessed any of these characteristics prior to the onset of the depression. If they indeed predisposed your teen to the current episode, they will certainly predispose her to a second episode. Enlisting the help of a therapist will do more than just bring your teenager a measure of peace and happiness; it may well prevent a recurrence.

Inadequate social support. Loss of social support may occur from the death of a parent, a divorce, suspension from high school, or flunking out of college. These situations will intensify the feelings of worthlessness and hopelessness that already plague the depressed teen. A skilled and experienced therapist can extricate the teen from much of the pain these situations cause. A more insidious way your teen's social support may erode is called distancing. You may become guilty of it when your teen's behavior turns obnoxious and then you "stay away" from him. It's more than rejection. It's the removal of all the support you provide via your encouragement and companionship. I was guilty of this with Eric. At times during his depression his behavior was so disagreeable that I would "leave him alone." I was tired of his irritability, and I was sure he was tired of me. But as I watched him suffer alone, I realized I had left him to fight his battle alone. That was unacceptable. My mistake gave me an understanding of the special peril facing parents with a depressed teen who also has oppositional-defiant disorder. This kind of teen's behavior seems constantly contrary to the family's values and expectations. It's no wonder, then, that Michelle's father was once moved to say, "When she goes to college, my only stipulation is that she goes far away." Michelle's father, too, knows he had frequently distanced himself from her. He made sure she had a therapist to talk to when the situation at home interfered with parental support.

Ongoing stress or adversity. Some things never go away. They seem unresolvable. Such was the tension inside Lauren's house because of festering marital discord. So, too, was the harassment Dan received at school because of his emerging homosexuality. Both of them attempted suicide more than once. Remember that a depressed teen is prone to collapse even under the continual pressure of normal stressors. You can then understand why psychologists speak of "the deadly triad." It's defined as a chronic stressor, loss of support, and hopelessness.

Finding Help for Your Teenager

If you think your teen meets any of the above criteria, request a referral to a mental health therapist. Be prepared to overcome some obstacles.

First, your doctor may shy away from the idea because she doesn't believe in psychotherapy. This would be surprising given all the studies that catalog its benefits, yet, in their hearts, many doctors doubt that psychotherapy works. This is largely a consequence of Freud and his quaint theories about the Oedipus complex, penis envy, and the like. What was all that about, anyway? Doctors like to know why things work, and the chemical mechanism of inhibition of serotonin reuptake appeals to the medical intellect. Also, drugs require less frequent and less intensive contact between patient and practitioner. Life for both the patient and the doctor is easier.

Second, psychotherapy doesn't come cheap. To get the typical twelve or twenty visits approved by your health insurer means an expenditure of several thousand dollars. As an advocate for your teenager, point out that if the extra short-term expense means a quicker recovery or prevention of a future episode, then the long-term expense will be less. In other words, psychotherapy will be cost-effective. Such effectiveness studies are in progress right now. Already, one conducted by Seattle's Group Health Cooperative has found that "the improved care of depression in primary care is a prudent investment of health care resources." If your health insurer needs this kind of convincing, ask your doctor to look up the most recently published studies on the National Library of Medicine's Web site (www.ncbi.nlm.nih.gov/PubMed). You can look them up yourself by using a combination of search words such as "depression combined psychotherapy cost."

Finally, even when you get a referral, there are relatively few therapists to go around, and they are overworked. "In my own practice," says Timothy Gibbs, M.D., president of the Minnesota Society for Child and Adolescent Psychiatry, "new patients almost always say they reached me after talking to two or three offices that were not accepting patients." There are only 6,700 board-certified child and adolescent psychiatrists in the country, and more practitioners are leaving the field than coming into it. The situation is not much better for child psychologists. "It's at least a four-month wait," says Jana Martin, Ph.D., past president of the California Psychological Association. "I'm booked solid." Psychiatric social workers who have experience with adolescents are also in short supply. "Availability is not good," recalls Lauren's mother. "It took a couple of months. It scared me. I was her parent, so I filled in the void in the health-care system."

Certainly, ask your teen's doctor to help find a psychotherapist. My own experience with Eric's primary care doctor, though, convinced me you also should be involved from the get-go, as Eric's doctor seemed disinterested in psychotherapy.

Ask other parents who are your friends for names. You'll be surprised how many of them will confide that their own teens have been depressed, and you will get candid firsthand evaluations. Ask the head of your religious congregation. Part of his regular counseling duties is to search out mental health therapists, especially those whose values coincide with those of his congregation. Ask the school psychologist or social worker to give you a list of competent therapists in your community who are experienced with teens. Then, take your list of names to your teen's doctor, add it to hers, and sort out the candidates together. You will need a lot of names. During the interviews for this book, I was surprised to learn how many teens and parents felt the need to switch therapists midstream, and more than once. It was more than half.

If your teen is ill enough to require a psychotherapist, he will probably need twelve to twenty visits. Unfortunately, the bias today is toward brief therapy—about three visits. It seems that the paradigms for depression shift only slowly. It took a long time to shift from the attitude that depression should be treated with exorcism or incarceration. It is also taking a long time to shift to the view that teen depression is not a self-limiting condition requiring only a short-term treatment. With this inaccurate perspective, psychotherapy would seem to be too complex a solution for such a simple problem. It is reassuring that doctors are coming to believe that teen depression is not simple at all. It is an illness with a high likelihood of recurrence, and sometimes it will become chronic, never remitting to anything better than a lifetime of agonizing dysthymia.

Nevertheless, your insurer might allow only three visits. What do you do when the insurance benefits run out? Sometimes, mental health professionals can justify the continuation of therapy and convince insurance companies to extend the benefits. Some therapists will offer "sliding scale" fees and continue therapy at reduced rates if you are paying out of pocket. Ask about this. In addition, make sure you read chapter 10 on the aspects of emotional therapy that you as a parent are capable of providing. You might have to be a stand-in for some disallowed visits.

What should you do if you have no health insurance or inadequate coverage? If you live in or near a city with a university or a medical school, teaching clinics often offer mental health services at reduced fees. The services are usually provided by students, but with faculty supervision. Also, religious organizations maintain rosters of therapists who will provide services on a sliding scale dictated by your income and the number of people in your family, with the fee as low as five dollars or sometimes even being waived. In Minneapolis, for example, Catholic Charities, Lutheran Social Services, and Jewish Family and Child Services have such rosters. Catholic Charities and Lutheran Social Services, in fact, maintain their own clinics with their own therapists, not only in Minneapolis and St. Paul but also in outlying rural areas. If your city has no such organization, contact your county's mental health department. If you aren't sure where to start, try calling 211 on your telephone. This number, First Call for Help, is managed by the United Way. In some states, your call will be routed to the appropriate social service agency in your area. It will help find you a counselor to fit your situation and income.

How to Choose a Therapist

Start by checking credentials. If your state requires licensure, make sure the therapist to whom your teen gets referred is indeed licensed. Five disciplines are recognized to care for patients with emotional illnesses.

A child and adolescent psychiatrist is a physician who obtains an M.D. degree and then receives specialty training in psychiatry. A child psychologist is not a physician but obtains a Ph.D. in counseling psychology, but a child psychologist cannot prescribe medications as can a psychiatrist.

Psychiatric nurses are recognized specialists, with some of them subspecializing in adolescent psychiatry. They obtain an R.N.

(registered nurse) designation. Not only do they counsel individual patients, but they may also be asked by managed care organizations to conduct psycho-educational classes for depressed adolescents and their families.

Social workers get a master's degree, or M.S.W., in their discipline. They have cared for persons with mental disorders ever since a psychiatric social worker, Elizabeth Horton, was appointed to the New York City hospital system in 1907.

Finally, marriage and family therapists, who obtain a master's degree or a Ph.D., make up a growing percentage of the mental health care force. "Five thousand of us specialize in adolescent depression," says Tony Jurich, Ph.D., past president of the American Association for Marriage and Family Therapy. "A lot of people don't see us in that role, because they focus on the first word—*marriage*."

Next, you want to ask the therapist which school or philosophy of psychotherapy she embraces. There are many schools of human behavior, but only three seem relevant:

- *Cognitive-behavioral therapy (CBT)* emphasizes that depression is something of a learned problem. The teen falls prey to the "negative triad," and the therapist tries to undo the teen's distorted thinking to alleviate the symptoms.
- *Interpersonal therapy (IPT)* focuses on problematic relationships in the teen's life. Eliminating interpersonal inadequacies or conflicts may eliminate some of the symptoms.
- *Family therapy (FT)* holds that teen mental health can be a reflection of family mental health. If all family members develop healthier interactions with one another, the depression should ease.

Although all three oversimplify the approach to depression, you want to make the closest possible match between your teen's particular problem and the therapeutic approach. After all, you have a good idea whether your teen's problems coincide with distorted thinking, difficult personal relationships, or a particularly dysfunctional family situation. "When you are living with it every day," Alison's father said, "it's always scattered out in front of you." Most therapists will reply that their approach is eclectic. It often doesn't work out that way in practice, however, because it is difficult for therapists to give up a bias learned in their early training.

Finally, ask the therapist if he specializes in adolescence and what kind of experience he has had treating depression. You may have to settle for someone with little experience with teens simply because the adolescent specialists are booked up for months.

Ask the therapist if he can give you data about past patients regarding their relapse rates and recurrence rates. If your teen has attempted, threatened, or seriously considered suicide, then suicide prevention is an item of prime concern. "Blake attempted suicide, and I was scared he would do it again," his mother said. "I asked the psychiatrist if any teenagers committed suicide while he was on watch. He said in thirty years of practice he never had one suicide. I sent Blake to him."

Once you are past these basic criteria, give your attention to other important considerations. Be picky about whom you choose. You are entrusting your teen to that person. "I had to have that lock-and-key fit," Lauren's mother said. Discussing the following items beforehand will help you determine if the therapist is a good fit.

Communication with your teen. Teenagers, more so the boys, don't like to talk about sensitive issues with adults, especially strange adults. On top of that, some depressed teens are volatile and react with tantrums, angry outbursts, or even destructive behavior when their issues come up for discussion. "She yelled she didn't want to talk to him because she didn't like him," Carla's mother said about her daughter's behavior in therapy. Lauren was luckier. "Her second therapist said things that really clicked for Lauren," her mother said. "She gave her strategies, gave her things to think about, went through scenarios with her. Lauren learned from her." Ask the therapist how he will get your teen to talk. To avoid detours in communication, make sure you tell him the issues about which your teen is especially prone to lie or withhold information. Eric would never tell how bad he felt.

Communication with you. You are the parent. This also makes you responsible. There's no arguing that you deserve regular communications from the therapist about what is happening in therapy. As a parental partner who intends to help your teenager, it's essential. Unfortunately, Eric's initial therapist didn't subscribe to this view. After a few sessions without a phone call, I asked for some feedback. I offered to meet the therapist at his convenience and pay him for his time. Even then, he gave it begrudgingly. Inevitably, he had to be let go. Make sure you ask how you can communicate information to the therapist and keep her updated. Your input is priceless. "Michelle's first therapist was great," her father said. "You could e-mail her anytime. She would e-mail you back in several hours max. That's necessary. With someone like Michelle, the situation can change rapidly. We also had our share of crises that demanded immediate attention." Don't be afraid to fire a therapist for poor communication. It's a deal-breaker.

Therapist's view of depression. It would seem in an enlightened information age that most or all therapists would have a scientific understanding of the three-part nature of depression: extrinsic factors such as chronic stress affect an intrinsically susceptible person who then experiences a change in brain chemistry. But not all therapists have this understanding. Eric's initial therapist saw only the stresses Eric experienced at home and at school and considered Eric a kind of victim of circumstances who needed to be rescued. But Eric also needed medicines. On the other hand, therapists can forget the stresses and get focused on the biology. "Carla said he didn't really want to know why she felt so bad today," her mother said. "He would tell her just to up her dosage. Even I know better. You have to get to the root of the problem."

Family values. "I searched for a credible physician whose goals were compatible with the goals of the family," Blake's mother said. For example, if you believe the family should be preserved at any reasonable cost, don't choose a therapist who believes it is readily disposable.

Family-based treatment. Does the therapist subscribe to the view that the family plays an important role in the teenager's recovery from depression? Explain the concept of parental partnering and gauge the therapist's reaction. It is counterproductive to choose a therapist who wants to exclude parents from the process.

"Quick fix" approach. "They've got labels," Michelle's father said. "They've got a quick fix because they have a pill that fits the label. Michelle was hard to figure out. How could [the therapist] figure it out so fast? It's been five years, and I'm still trying to figure Michelle out. It's not right, but they do that because they are too busy and overworked." Michelle's father was absolutely correct. The acute shortage of therapists in America today, and the often abbreviated treatment schedules insurers allow, may get your teenager a "production line" approach. Always question the therapist about a diagnosis or impression that you don't understand or strikes you as off-base. Doctors use the term *working diagnosis* to mean "I'm not sure what this illness is, but this is what I'm going to call it until something happens to make me change my mind." If that's the best that can be done, it's okay to have a working diagnosis. Just make sure you know what it is.

Skills. You may feel that your teen has difficulty with self-control, relaxation, interpersonal relationships, or negative thoughts. Ask the therapist if she will teach remedial skills, and whether she will give your teen related homework. "The negative thinking has to be challenged constantly," Katie's mother said. Skills are most important, because a depressed teen must develop self-efficacy. During one of our "serious" conversations, Eric pointed out the need for self-efficacy so well: "Why was this school so different the day before? Who touched me? What did I say? What did I do the day before to feel so good?" He yearned to know what to do.

Hospitalization. If your teen is seriously ill, ask the therapist for her views on hospitalizing him. When a real danger of suicide arises, hospitalization seems mandatory to preserve a life. However, for lesser crises such as emotional outbursts, some therapists rightly feel that hospitalization disempowers the family. Figure out with the therapist how the issue of disempowerment fits into your situation and values.

Fees. Clarify what the therapist charges for each session, and how his office handles health insurance claims. If insurance will not cover any or enough therapy sessions, ask if there is a sliding-scale option.

Session length and session schedule. Some teenagers will talk, but they may not be able to do it productively during a fifty-minute hour. Ask the therapist if she will consider shorter and more frequent sessions in this case.

Group therapy. This is another way a therapist may get a poorly communicative teen to talk. A group of peers may be less intimidating than a strange adult. Yet, this may not be to your liking, particularly with comorbid anorexia nervosa. "I wanted to avoid a group situation," Katie's mother said. "I didn't want this to become part of Katie's identity, as how she saw herself."

Parent education. If you intend to help, or if you intend to correct any contribution you may be making to the depression, you will need to learn about your teen's diagnoses. This is called psychoeducation. Make sure the therapist offers it or at least gives you a list of sources of information.

Psychometrics. Many psychology companies publish symptom-rating scales for depression and most comorbid conditions. (They even publish one for fear of spiders.) Ask the therapist if she will use these to measure the severity of the depression and other illnesses both at the beginning and the end of treatment. If not, ask her how she will judge whether your teen has made sufficient progress to stop treatment and to avoid a relapse or recurrence.

Concluding Therapy

At the end of treatment, the therapist should give you and your teen a to-do list tailored to your teen's emotional problems. Don't leave without it. No matter how good the treatment was, the chances of recurrence remain high. The to-do list will help you with your ongoing role as your teenager's cotherapist at home.

How will you know when it's time to terminate your teen's therapy? Don't expect the therapist to tell you. While many therapists have a balanced perspective on termination, some encourage their clients to continue longer than necessary. As the parental partner, you, along with your teenager, need to decide when enough talk is enough. Do your detective work. Three months of therapy is a good benchmark. Ask your teenager if he wants to continue. Does he think he can cope without therapy? Does he feel that he has more to express, explore, and learn—or does he think that he and the therapist have covered most bases? Does he feel his depression has subsided? Review the symptom chart in chapter 7 together and see how he's progressing. You'll have to use a combination of investigation, intuition, and common sense to decide when to wrap up therapy.

Another option is to taper off. Some therapists will see a client biweekly, or even once a month. Also ask about periodic booster sessions after the completion of regular therapy. Some preliminary studies indicate they may help prevent recurrences of the depression.

Questions to Ask When Interviewing a Therapist

- What are your credentials? Are you licensed?
- What type of therapy do you do? (cognitive-behavioral, interpersonal, etc.)
- How much experience have you had with teenagers?
- Do you have data on the relapse and recovery rates of your clients who suffer from depression?
- What are your fees? Do you accept our type of health insurance? Do you offer a sliding scale if we have to pay out of pocket?
- When are you available to start seeing my teenager?
- Is there flexibility regarding session length and schedule?
- How do you feel about medication combined with therapy for depression?
- What is your experience with suicidal patients? What are your views on hospitalization if there is a risk of suicide?
- What methods do you use to break through communication barriers with teenagers?
- Are you willing to keep me regularly informed about the progress of the therapy?
- How do you feel about family-based therapy and the idea of parental partnering?
- Do you have any special beliefs on religious or family values that we need to discuss?
- How do you measure the teenager's progress?
- How do you decide when it's time to stop therapy? Do you offer booster sessions?

9

Strategy Seven
Take the Family Inventory

Dr. Emmy Werner was surprised to find herself far away on the island of Kauai designing advertisements for milk cartons. She had just gotten her Ph.D. in child psychology from the University of Nebraska, and now she was over three thousand miles west of Lincoln, on the end of the Hawaiian archipelago. Surprised, yes, but she felt excited she could now embark on the kind of study that was rarely attempted because of its presumed impossibility.

It was 1955, and psychologists hadn't yet decided to dissect human behavior into minute traits with antiseptic academic labels. Instead, Dr. Werner was looking at the big picture. She also made sure she didn't forget the humanistic aspect of life. The point of her study was to ask a simple and fundamental question: Does an emotionally unhealthy family produce emotionally unhealthy children? To get an answer, though, Dr. Werner needed a group of subjects she could study for decades after they were born. But that kind of follow-up usually was impossible. To solve the problem, she would go to Kauai. Historically, mobility there was limited. People born on Kauai tended to stay on Kauai. Moreover, the population of the island was markedly heterogeneous, with children of diverse cultural backgrounds—Japanese, Korean, Filipino, Portuguese, Chinese, northern European, and, of course, Hawaiian. To make the study's results widely relevant, she wanted it to embrace many kinds of children.

She set to work publicizing her study with announcements at women's groups, church gatherings, and, yes, even with advertisements on the sides of milk cartons. Eventually, she got to study every baby born on Kauai in 1955, all 698 of them. Her plan ultimately worked, and she succeeded in keeping track of 80 percent of the study's surviving subjects even thirty years later.

Dr. Werner's common sense proved true. When the family was not emotionally healthy, the added stress of family dysfunction often made for an unhappy outcome. In fact, Dr. Werner had initially identified 201 of Kauai's newborn children that year as being at risk because of "adverse rearing conditions" such as poverty, desertion, parental discord, or parental alcoholism. Years into the study, two-thirds of them had delinquency records, learning or behavioral problems, or unwanted pregnancies. Seventy of these children at risk eventually developed an emotional illness, oftentimes depression.

Just as Dr. Werner took inventory of Kauai's families to look for significant dysfunctional characteristics, so, too, should you take inventory of your own family. You'll probably find some dysfunctions that could be promoting your teen's depression. I certainly did in mine. I still chuckle every time I think of the old quip about holding a "functional families" convention—and no one shows up. It gets me off the defensive when it comes time to take my periodic inventory and check for improvement. My family will never be perfect, and I don't think we'll be going to that convention anytime soon.

The point of the family inventory is not to do an attic-to-basement housecleaning. That's unrealistic. The point of the inventory is to shift the balance. You want to cultivate a family climate of positive qualities—and prune back the bad ones. "I have no fear of questioning where I went wrong," Dan's mother said. "I question and question and question. The trouble is that I'm much more certain in my professional life than my family life." By identifying and fixing as many stress-producing family characteristics as is reasonable, you might shift the balance in your teen's favor, and that may be sufficient.

Family Climate

Scientific investigations into the biology of depression have occupied center stage for nearly two decades. Now, thankfully, the interpersonal relationships of depressed people are again becoming a focus for psychological research into the causes and outcome of depressive illness. In fact, many of the most recently reported findings repeat that teen depression is related to the levels of support, attachment, and approval provided by the family. After all, for a teen, the most important interpersonal relationships are within the family, especially with parents. The climate the family creates is a major influence on a teen's mood. The better the mental health of the family is, the less likely will its sons and daughters develop depression. And if they do get depressed because of an inescapable susceptibility, the course of the depression should be milder. You want to check that your family has high levels of those certain qualities that can counter depression.

When I was a first-year medical student at the University of

Michigan, I learned right away that doctors could be classified as either "lumpers" or "splitters." For the splitters, no medical problem is simple, but represents a variant of a broader condition, and the variant needs to be considered in all its minor details to distinguish it from all the other variants. The lumpers, however, take the overview, hoping they can discern some generalizable truth by not getting distracted with the details. It's the reason surgeons, in facetiously distinguishing themselves from the professedly more "cerebral" internists, poke fun at themselves by saying, "We don't know many of the details, but we can certainly help you." The lumpers watch the forest. The splitters watch the trees.

When it comes to the health of the family, I want to be a lumper. I don't want to get bogged down with a plethora of scientific studies that examine the hundreds of minifacets or microtraits now alleged to define the family climate. I want the big picture, because that is the only practical way I can deal with my family. I don't really know how to examine for and correct a lack of "microsocialization triumphs," for example, especially when the study's findings are couched in "scree plots" and "orthogonal rotations." I do know, however, when my son doesn't feel good about himself and when my family may not be working to turn that around. I know because it's part of my nature as a parent.

For the family with a depressed adolescent, I distilled four crucial human elements necessary for a beneficial family climate. Identifying these elements required not only thinking about the qualities that are important in my family, but also reviewing the hundred or so parent interviews I conducted for this book. I looked for the common threads, derived from parent wisdom. In the end, four essential family attributes emerged:

- Belonging
- Respect for autonomy

- Self-esteem
- Intimacy

Each attribute is broad. Each contains loads of that mini- and micro-stuff written in scholarly journals. And each overlaps with its three partners. You may lump these qualities a bit differently for your depressed teen. However, in the final analysis, we'll be talking about the same attributes. An inventory of how these qualities are represented in your family may help you identify possible underlying causes of your teenager's depression.

Your teen's sense of belonging within the family. Human beings crave interpersonal bonds. These provide security, sustenance, companionship, and well-being. A matchless bond is forged for the teen when the family values her involvement, and when the family communicates that she "fits" well in the family. This kind of bond proclaims to her a genuine sense of belonging. Belonging gives the teen a feeling of meaningfulness and establishes for her a viable base that positively shapes her behavior and emotions. When a vulnerable teen doesn't feel she belongs, any chronic stressor that can trigger or promote depression is much less bearable.

How strong the sense of belonging is determines the answer to a question of critical importance to any adolescent, especially the one who is doubting her self-worth while in the throes of depression: "How much do I matter to this family?" Chloe was an art student and didn't think she mattered much to her father because he didn't value her kind of involvement. She hungered for the worth that eluded her and tried to solve the problem by adopting his hobbies. "I learned to do the activities he liked. I convinced him I could work on a car. I did a brake job all by myself. It took me three nights, and I had to read a lot of books. But I did it. I got pretty good in his woodworking shop, too."

Jared's ADHD was a terrible obstacle to belonging. "I guess he didn't fit," said Jared's mother. "Sometimes when [his sister] would have friends over, he would pick on them and put on a disastrous show. This went beyond the usual 'brother thing' because he didn't know when to quit. We've really had to work accepting Jared for [who] he is."

Certain basic factors foster the teen's sense of belonging to the family. Affection, acceptance, and supportive interactions with the teen are the central elements. They announce loud and clear that the teen's involvement in the family is highly valued. Be careful, though, since an overdose of support may morph into overprotection. This diminishes a teen's sense of belonging because an overprotective parenting style may be tantamount to control, and control implies that the teen is incompetent or may not fit so well.

High levels of conflict in parent-teen relationships similarly point to a poor fit, and the teen's perceived sense of belonging dwindles. Lauren's mother said it this way: "The attachments with her had always been fractured. There was one black shoe among all the brown shoes." Of course, abusive interactions are malignant. They obliterate the sense of belonging. When the teen feels little sense of belonging to the family, the result is loneliness, and loneliness is associated with worse depression and with more frequent thoughts of suicide.

The family's sense of belonging within the community. A large survey of Alameda County, California, residents thirty years ago proved that the more friends and acquaintances you had, the more volunteer and religious organizations you belonged to, the lower were the rates of death and disease you would experience. Getting more involved in the community actually made the family healthier and its members were less depressed. The reason was more than just better access to the community's social and material resources. Being strongly connected to the community allowed the family to learn its strategies, its social norms, for physical and emotional well-being. Moreover, community involvement made social loneliness impossible.

Years later, researchers put the issue to a scientific test by studying people who had suffered brain injuries from automobile or motorcycle accidents. These individuals had experienced significant nervous system trauma, with a learning disability or paralysis resulting. To various degrees, these problems cut them off from friends and organizations within the community. The study's results showed a second injury: for most of these injured people, a decreased sense of belonging to the community reliably predicted their postinjury depression.

Teenagers whose families lack strong social relationships within the community are more vulnerable to depression. "In high school I felt lonely a lot," Chloe said. "My father is bipolar, and my brother is schizophrenic. My family was weird. They were pretty isolated, and they never got involved outside. They never went to church. They never had many friends. At times I felt suffocated by them."

The community itself may be a part of the problem. It may have poorly developed social resources such as parks or recreational facilities. Or, as may happen in a rural community, it may be isolated from geographically distant resources. A common complaint among teenagers is that "there's nothing to do in this town," and sometimes it's true. Perhaps your family doesn't feel comfortable in the community because of socioeconomic, religious, or political differences. You have to weigh these factors as a parent-partner. A depressed teen is such an ill person that a change of community, though difficult, may be a prescription to consider.

Respect for your teen's developing autonomy. When your teen was a young child, the power relationship between the two of you was markedly asymmetric. In essence, you were a benevolent dictator. Adolescence, however, spurs your teen to renegotiate her power relationship with you into a more balanced state of affairs. Now, you must ratchet down from dictator to consultant. Your parenting style must change from authoritarian to authoritative. If, however, it remains autocratic, and the teen is not allowed more input into decision-making, the consequences can be severe. This kind of rigidity prevents your teen from learning problem-solving strategies and coping skills, two assets crucial for preventing and combating depression.

Teen self-esteem. Perhaps you are tired of hearing the hackneyed term *self-esteem* because it's been bantered about so casually and so long for adult problems everywhere from the workplace to the golf course. Rest assured, though, it is a big deal for teens, because the enormous physical and intellectual changes they are undergoing generate doubts and insecurities about the self daily. It is wise to heed psychiatrist Harold Koplewicz's pronouncement that "for many teens, inadequacy is the salient sentiment of these years." After all, they are learning new physical and mental skills, but have usually mastered few of them. They are moving in new social groups, and usually feel awkward and uncomfortable. All the while, their actions are visible to the "imaginary audience," as psychologist David Elkind calls it. They think they are constantly on display and that others are always scrutinizing them, although in reality seldom is anyone taking notes. Thus, when an insult to a teen's self-esteem occurs, it often gets inflated and hits the teen hard because of his intellectual immaturity. Just consider what happens when acne strikes. Doctors know that most teenagers overestimate the severity of the problem and consider it a cataclysm.

Under constant and intense self-criticism, a teen with little self-esteem is easy prey for depression. If the teen is already depressed, damaged self-esteem shackles him with self-loathing. "[My husband] and I are both perfectionists," Jared's mother said. "Jared lacks motivation and wasn't studying. He wasn't making good grades. Then there would be that critical talk that was very damaging. I had to let it go. I had to remind myself he was depressed."

For this reason, too, Chloe suffered a recurrence of her depression in college. "I'm tripping myself up with my low self-esteem. It gets in the way of my dating and making new friends. Part of me really wants to be noticed, but because I was afraid, I would make people come to me. They thought I was aloof. Everybody else is dating and getting married. I feel I'm behind. I don't know what to do."

Promoting healthy self-esteem in your teen confers particular advantages to combat depression. It allows your teen to discriminate between relevant and irrelevant information, reduces susceptibility to ephemeral events, and increases the perception of one's self-efficacy, all potent weapons against worthlessness and hopelessness. Your teen needs a healthy estimate of her own self-worth. She must be able to say to herself, as much as possible, "I'm confident, happy, competitive, ambitious, hardworking, good-looking, good in sports, creative, independent, honest, generous, caring, expressive, outgoing, and good at schoolwork."

The parent has the unique capacity to be a teen's biggest booster. Of course, your teenager might not accept your praise graciously, or at all. She may give you evidence that contradicts every compliment. Nevertheless, although your words are denied, they are being heard—and they help.

Intimacy. The best definition I've encountered for family intimacy is "loving companionship." We long for this kind of interpersonal relationship in which we can dismiss the pretenses, expose our vulnerabilities without fear, and have the substance of our selves welcomed into the life of another person. We reciprocate in kind. Then, the two of us are no longer strangers. We are connected. With a bit of luck, we will become soul mates.

Loss of intimacy is a loss of the first order. It's no wonder, then, that adolescents who wind up depressed have experienced less intimacy with their parents. Challenges to intimacy occur in any relationship because, by definition, relationships are always in flux. They certainly occur in any family, because families always have conflicts.

And conflicts often flare up in adolescence. But "I disagree with you" shouldn't mean I dislike you, disrespect you, or want to distance myself from you.

In addition, challenges to intimacy occur because our postmodern lifestyle encourages materialism and anonymity. Parents may be too busy working to engage in the relaxed, day-to-day conversation that fosters intimacy. Teenagers are swayed by pop culture to cluster with their peers and exclude their parents. A gigantic challenge is parental divorce, where the intimacy of the father-child relationship suffers more than that of the mother-child one in most cases.

Even in families that stay together, father-daughter intimacy often suffers during the teenage years. It's jarring when sweet little girls develop into moody young women. Fathers may react to their discomfort by becoming more distant. The gulf widens when teenage girls become enmeshed in their Byzantine social lives and perhaps abandon the sports and interests they once shared with their fathers.

These challenges are difficult, but they can't be allowed to undermine intimacy. Closeness with your teen is too valuable in the fight against depression, and feels too good, to let anything get in the way.

Family Stress

What family can ever escape stress? With a depressed teen, the idea is to identify the stress promptly and then intervene. If you are able to reduce the stress, you can change the balance in your teen's favor. Review the following list of stressors that spring from family circumstances and are known to promote teen depression. If any of them apply to you, bring them up with your teen's physician. Defy the statistics that show most families conceal problematic family relationships and difficult family circumstances from their physician.

Interparental conflict. This kind of conflict is dangerous to your teen's mental health. It promotes aggression, conduct problems, antisocial behavior, anxiety, withdrawal, and depression. If you and your spouse can't resolve your issues, then try to implement some protective buffers against the chronic stress it causes for your teen. First, make sure your teen feels a strong sense of parental attachment. This communicates that the family will continue to be a source of stability and support despite the obvious disruption of interparental relationships. Intimacy with either or both parents seems effective in overcoming the negative effects of the conflict. Second, make sure parental monitoring and supervision continue unabated. This tells the teen loudly that the parents nevertheless remain involved and interested in his well-being. Finally, encourage strong and healthy peer relationships. These may provide reassurance that an alternative source exists to meet some of your teen's emotional needs when they can't be met at home in the family.

Divorce. After thirty years of scientific debate, there still is no scientific consensus emerging on how parental divorce influences the emotional well-being of teens. But it doesn't take a scientist to figure out that divorce can be a double whammy for teenagers who are susceptible to depression. First of all, divorce may set off a chain of stresses such as litigation, relocation, custody disagreements, and economic hardship. Daily life may become somewhat unstructured or even chaotic. Second, divorce diminishes the teen's ability to deal with the stresses. The teen's socialization environment is disrupted. Parental support diminishes as parental influence erodes. The situation worsens substantially if economic hardship ensues. Divorce is a common and frequently forgotten cause for a dramatic decline in the family's standard of living, with many female-headed families falling into poverty.

Stepfamilies. Among teens, emotional problems, including depression, increase in families where children reside with stepmothers, but not so much in stepfather families. The facts are firm, but the reasons are conjectural. Perhaps the loss of the biological mother is somehow more significant than the loss of the biological father. Or perhaps the biological mother did not win custody of the children because she was abusive, addicted, or irresponsible, and the effects of past maternal abuse continue to manifest themselves later, even with a benevolent and loving stepmother.

Parental depression. Teen depression often follows parental depression. It's more than genes, and the additional reasons are legion. For instance, depressed parents are less intimate with their teens, withdraw from them, and provide less care. "My depression worsens every fall," said Jared's mother. "I might be dysthymic. It alters my thinking. I might not have enough energy for Jared. I do what I have to do, but there is a lack of excitement." Then, too, depressed parents may "teach" their children depression. Jared's mother went on to say, "I may teach Jared depressed ways of thinking. He was bullied and didn't do well on the school bus. At one point then, I was enabling him to be a victim. Jared was always a victim."

Dan's depressed mother was eloquent in her warning: "My own problems were transferred to Dan. We should be aware of our own vulnerabilities and foibles. If you see it in your child and it is a problem, look to see if it is in you."

Economic hardship. Psychological problems, especially depression, are more prevalent and of greater severity among poorer teens. Economically disadvantaged families experience more adverse and stressful life events such as frequent moves, overcrowding, and increased parental conflict. This causes teens in low-income families to feel a reduced sense of control and mastery over material conditions and, consequently, an ineffectiveness over their own personal problems. If depression strikes, it exacerbates an already established sense of hopelessness.

Acculturative stress. Studies have shown that migrant farm-workers and their children experience more anxiety and depression.

The combination of possible family dysfunction, low self-esteem, and economic hardship can be crushing. Many diverse groups suffer from this syndrome. Here in Minneapolis we have the largest Hmong population in the United States. Psychiatrists see a disproportionate number of depressed teenagers from this community.

Witnessing community violence. This applies especially to males, ethnic minorities, and urban residents. The risk for depression increases especially in the presence of family conflict or family violence on top of community violence.

Family Pathology

The following are the extreme stressors. They are inexcusable and must stop. If any of these pathologies are present in your family, seek help without delay.

Parental addiction. The addicted parent is often wrapped up in his own problems and has little time for the teen's. Moreover, when intoxicated, a parent is unavailable to a teenager who may be in crisis. "For most of his life, her father didn't eat dinner with us," Chloe's mother said. "He would prefer eating in the basement in front of the TV and drinking beer. By nine o'clock he had a pretty good buzz on." According to authoritative estimates, up to 30 percent of American families have an addicted parent. Thankfully, a wide network of organizations based on the twelve-step program of Alcoholics Anonymous can help. For information about groups in your area, check your local telephone directory or log on to www.alcoholics-anonymous.org (for alcohol abuse) or www.na.org (for drug addiction). Family members who are affected by alcoholism or substance abuse can turn to Al-Anon/Alateen, which can be reached at 888-4AL-ANON or www.al-anon.alateen.org.

Sexual abuse. Parental sexual abuse promotes depression and accelerates its onset in both teenage girls and boys. In addition, these teens experience more aggression, substance abuse, and sexual risk-taking. Sexual abuse of a teenager by someone outside the family is also a serious threat to the teenager's emotional health. It must be confronted and stopped immediately.

Physical abuse. With almost 1 million cases of adolescent abuse and neglect reported in the United States each year, maltreatment of teens is an urgent national problem. Adolescence encourages parent-child conflict. A lot of adolescent behavior can annoy or provoke parents. Because of their immaturity, teens have difficulty controlling their behavior, conforming to standards the family has established, or achieving assigned tasks. Because of their own "middle-age" developmental stage, parents may find themselves at loggerheads with their own teens. The parent's sexuality may be declining as the teen's is emerging. A parent's energy may be waning as the teen's is building. All of this sets the stage for a parent who lacks management skills. It's no wonder, then, that a "disciplinary measure" becomes overly punitive. Spanking with the hand may evolve into striking with a fist, belt, or worse. It is surprising, though, that most abusers of teens are mothers or maternal figures. Adolescent abuse leads to depression, generalized anxiety disorder, and an overall sense of dependency and helplessness. If you need help to curb abuse in your family, contact Parents Anonymous. This respected national organization provides weekly support groups and educational groups free of charge. For a meeting in your area, log on to www.parentsanonymous.org.

Verbal abuse. Many parents don't realize that verbal abuse is a family pathology, and one of the most insidious. Sometimes it's called emotional abuse or verbal violence. Whatever you want to call it, it's a basic lack of human kindness. We often forget that words are just as harmful as actions. Belittling a teen with words causes suffering, too. Abusive words diminish the teen's self-esteem and invalidate his feelings. When the abusive language comes from a parent, it stings the most. "I think we called him a *jerk* a few times," Jared's mother said. "And that was mild for what we were feeling. We called him *lazy,* too. Verbal abuse is major. It's very damaging. Our brains store up all this stuff we've heard. When you've heard it two or three times, it becomes a tape that keeps playing. This was what I dealt with all my life. My mom cut me down anytime she could."

Dan's mother became just as watchful as Jared's. "I had to be very cautious about what message I was sending," she said. "He responds to me. He takes my lead." Don't forget that an icy silence is also verbal abuse. It is easy to become verbally abusive when your teen demonstrates bad behavior such as truancy, drug usage, persistent curfew violations, running away, or socializing with "problem" friends. If verbal abuse is an issue in your family, contact Because I Love You, a national organization that provides parent support groups in over twenty-one states now. Log on to their Web site at www.becauseiloveyou.org.

Family Therapy

A family may face complex, multiple problems. When this happens, a therapeutic focus that includes only the teen may be too narrow, and a therapist may need to deal with the full ecology of the family. After all, the family represents the major stage on which a teenager deals with the depression. Perhaps you need to resurrect all the harmonious and helpful relationships that characterized your family before the depression set in. Also, the disruptive behavior that is so common with teen depression may have contaminated all of family life, with the result that new dysfunctions may have arisen in the family. In sum, a family with a depressed teen may find itself woefully short on interpersonal assets.

If you believe that the family is significantly dysfunctional and needs to be brought back into equilibrium, ask your physician about family therapy. Or if your teen is already seeing a psychotherapist, ask her if she has unearthed any problems that should be dealt with in family therapy.

Addressing covert family problems is one of the main goals of family therapy. For example, one parent may have formed an alliance with the teen against the other. Or a parent, often the mother, may be an enabler and "supplier" of an addicted teen. The problems may be more subtle, such as one parent denying the teenager's depression or blaming the other parent for it. In family therapy the parent is essentially asked for an examination of conscience. The question is put forth to the parent, "How did you contribute to the dysfunction in this family?"

You have to get to work right away. Family stresses predict relapses and recurrences of your teen's depression. You want this current depressive episode to disappear, and family therapy may be the best route. Here are some questions for you to consider. If you answer yes to any of them, family therapy should seriously be considered:

- Is your family concealing a major dysfunction such as abuse?
- Is communication within the family severely inadequate?
- Is your family plagued with stressful conflicts that have not been confronted?
- Does your teen have a conduct disorder or an eating disorder?
- Does your teen abuse drugs or alcohol?
- Does your family have an alcoholic identity, with several addicted persons and with alcohol or substance abuse being an organizing principle of the family?

You may have to swallow your pride to ask your teen's physician about the advisability of family therapy. The payoff, however, should be worth it. "We've been to quite a few family therapists," Jared's mother said. "It was an eye-opener to learn that Jared was manipulative. [My husband], Jared, and I were a triangle. Jared did what he wanted, and [my husband] and I would argue about it. We needed to work on how we would all interact. It was the best advice we ever got."

Family therapy has many potential benefits. It can:

- Empower the family
- Mobilize the intrinsic resources of the family
- Recruit both parents to advocate for their teen, if they are not doing it already
- Help to restructure bad relationships among family members by forcing them to confront and discuss their conflicts
- Counteract any negative influences from antisocial peers
- Teach families problem-solving skills

Family therapy is already proving its usefulness in certain situations. It reduces recurrences of schizophrenia and depression, and it appears effective in preventing the "transmission" of alcoholism to the family's next generation. If balance in the family is restored, it can resume its function as a nurturing center for its young adolescents and as a launching center for its older ones. Even if you don't see this kind of huge effect, family therapy may still be a genuine success. It may prevent your teen's treatment from being sabotaged by family dysfunctions.

Forgiveness

The pastor of my family's church is wise about sermons. For one thing, he makes them short. He also seems convinced that if the congregation goes away with one clear and memorable point that can be put into a few simple words, then his sermon is a resounding success. In his sermon two Sundays ago, he spoke about hurtful human relationships. He quoted an old and dear friend of his, a child and adolescent psychiatrist in suburban Minneapolis, Dr. Carl Hansen, with whom he had recently had lunch. He had asked the psychiatrist whether there was one reason above all to explain failures in psychotherapy with depressed teens. With almost thirty years' experience, Dr. Hansen didn't have to think twice for an answer: "Of course. It is lack of forgiveness. The teenager fails to forgive himself, or to forgive those who may have wronged him." It was a clear and memorable point.

It was also an intriguing answer because Dr. Hansen was explaining a medical failure not in clinical terms but in human ones. I called Monday morning and asked whether I might interview him at his office. The diplomas and certificates on its walls said he had received his M.D. from the University of Minnesota Medical School. Afterward, he trained as a child and adolescent psychiatrist at Yale from 1982 to 1984. Here's what we discussed.

Q. *Let me check my definition of forgiveness with you to make sure we're talking about the same thing. I understand it to mean letting go of negative emotions, thoughts, and behavior towards the wrongdoer, things like hostility, revenge, and any kind of aggression.*

A. Yes, that's right.

Q. *Does forgiveness include condoning the bad behavior or reconciliation with the wrongdoer, or even forgetting that the whole bad situation ever happened?*

A. Not at all. None of those things. Actually, reconciliation may be impossible because the wrongdoer might remain a dangerous individual.

Q. *Is lack of forgiveness a big deal?*

A. Lack of forgiveness is one of the greatest causes of failure in the treatment of teen depression. For example, in my practice I have had a number of depressed adolescent girls who attempted suicide after being rejected by a boy. These girls haven't forgiven themselves for not being able to make the relationship work. But lots of times it wasn't a good relationship anyway. Sometimes the boy was unfaithful or put a lot of pressure on her to have sex, drink, or use chemicals. He could pressure her a lot so she would avoid being with her family instead of with him. I also remember a young, depressed woman who couldn't improve until she forgave her sexually abusive father. She struggled from childhood on with suicide urges and attempts. She had no time free of depression until she forgave him. It dramatically reduced her anxiety and preoccupation with revenge. She even could maintain a distant relationship with him.

Q. *How does lack of forgiveness make depression worse?*

A. It causes rumination and guilt. It causes people to agonize over their life. People don't let go of things so the depression always percolates back up to the surface. Bad experiences repeat themselves without forgiveness.

Q. *How does lack of forgiveness interfere with recovery from depression?*

A. Experiences [from] people's pasts become an organizing factor for the present. When you face things square on, then you can master them. Otherwise, the situation in which you were wronged may become a compass for your life. There are better compasses. In teen depression, revenge is a big problem. They feel their situation is someone else's doing. I've seen teens who can't find revenge [who] will then attempt suicide.

Q. *How can a depressed teen achieve forgiveness?*

A. A lot of therapists run forgiveness groups to forgive abusive or addicted people. They ask the wronged person in the group to make up a grudge list in order to bring some of the repressed and unspoken hurts into consciousness. They'll do role-playing or reenactments so that the person can learn how to finally talk to the wrongdoer. For the same reason, the therapist might ask the person to write a letter to the wrongdoer. Seldom is it actually delivered. It can backfire because a wrongdoer may not want to take ownership of the problem. I believe the roots of forgiveness come out of the spiritual tradition. We recognize that we and others are imperfect. A wronged person can also find forgiveness with a [religious minister] or during a religious service centering on forgiveness.

Many depressed teens believe they have been wronged. In fact, depressed teens often are aversive to people and feel they have been victimized by them. You may need to convince your teenager that forgiveness could be an important part of her recovery. It might be an ex-boyfriend or ex-girlfriend your teenager has to forgive. Or someone closer to home. After you take the family inventory in this chapter, you might identify yourself as something of a wrongdoer. If that is the case, you might have to ask your teenager for forgiveness in order for her to move on.

Forgiveness is a two-way street. A depressed teenager can behave badly, too. You might be angry at certain behaviors or disappointed with perceived failures and shortcomings. If this is the situation, offer your teenager your forgiveness. Then you can continue as allies.

10

Strategy Eight
Bring the "Talking Cure" Home

Scientific journals are loaded with solid evidence that talk therapy is highly effective against depression. But one fifty-minute session each week for twelve weeks, or one twenty-minute session each week for twenty weeks, may be insufficient to undo a depressed teenager's faulty thinking habits. As a parent-partner you should consider taking on the awesome task of being a "cotherapist" at home. This does not mean that you can or should try to replace the skilled work of a professional therapist. But without realizing it, anytime you spoke to your depressed teen in the privacy of the home about how she views the world and what she thinks of herself, you were actually a cotherapist. You're not replacing her therapist. You're adding to the therapist's efforts. Don't worry about not having a counseling degree. You have other substantial qualifications—love and logic.

There are compelling reasons for you, as parent-partner, to assume some of the responsibility for correcting your teen's erroneous thinking. You have more contact with her than the short twenty-five or fifty minutes that the psychotherapist has available every week or so. You know quite well what many of her faulty thinking patterns are already without needing weeks or months of therapy to ferret them out. You know best how to correct her information-processing distortions, especially those that involve her negative self-evaluations. Finally, the task may default to you anyway, because your health insurer may cut the office-therapy visits short. Never forget that a parent is the most influential person to convince a depressed teen that there are other and better ways of seeing things. You have immense power to steer your teen's thinking back onto a true course and invigorate her interior life.

There are two requirements to become an effective cotherapist. First, you must be a good listener. You may not yet have gotten used to doing that with your child. After all, when she was younger, out of necessity, you were a benevolent dictator. You did a lot of the talking and she did a lot of the listening. Now that she is a teen, you must revamp your parental job description and transform yourself into a knowledgeable consultant. A good consultant is first a good listener. That old hierarchy of parent-then-child was clearly necessary. But hierarchy emphasizes distance. Now, that steep hierarchy must get leveled out a lot. It must give way to a relationship with more closeness in order to facilitate dialogue. Closeness combats depression's sense of worthlessness and hopelessness.

The second requirement of an effective cotherapist is that you must know how to talk to a depressed teenager. That may not be easy if your teen is reluctant to talk about uncomfortable issues or is just plain reticent. Worse yet, the lines of communication may be blocked by anger, resentment, lies, or denial. Don't worry. The insights and wisdom of other parents with depressed teens will come to the rescue.

Talking to Your Teen

Talking to a teenager is like "working a room." Just ask any comedian, motivational speaker, or cleric about this fearsome proposition. Jokes mysteriously fall flat. Seemingly innocuous comments can incite a chorus of boos. A person or two in the audience may fall asleep—and snore, too. If you are severely out of line, whether you think so or not, someone heaves a tomato. Talking to your teen is hazardous duty for a parent, yet there is no hazardous-duty pay.

Talking to a teenager is also one of a parent's most rewarding and endearing experiences. The success is all in the approach. A parent shouldn't try to be a proselytizing preacher or a mere cheerleader peddling hackneyed slogans. What the parent is during those warm and caring times of talking, sometimes late at night or sometimes after a good cry, is a teacher. No teacher pretends to have all the answers. No teacher believes his advice disallows other options. No teacher is brash or conceited. The parent who is a real teacher teaches from experience. Oftentimes, the first fine words out are "I've made this mistake. Here's what I learned so I could avoid it the next time." It's a humbling statement. But it's sincere, and it connects. Most of all, a teacher doesn't bluster, overawe, or intimidate. Rather, a teacher convinces, and I like to think of the parent-teacher as the preeminent convincer. Every day, essentially, a parent who is an effective teacher for his children will be saying, "Please, listen. There is some truth here. Weigh the evidence. I hope you might be persuaded."

To help you work the room of a teenager's mind, I've compiled a list of eleven dos and ten don'ts. This endeavor seems audacious, since bookstore shelves house lengthy volumes on the mysterious art of talking to a teen. I place a lot of faith in this list, though, because it is distilled from the parent interviews I conducted for this book. It's far from complete because each depressed teenager is unique and these parents are speaking specifically about their own experience.

But since the suggestions derive from parent wisdom, many should hold true for any of our teens.

Eleven Dos for Talking with Your Teen

1. Pay attention to timing. Alison's stepfather discovered what every worried parent does to create an opportunity for a heart-to-heart talk with a teenager. "Using the car gives you a captive audience. Alison was in cheerleading, and so it was a twenty-minute drive when I picked her up. She couldn't head for the bathroom." "Driving is a very good time," Heidi's mother said. "I used to pick her up every day. It was twenty minutes of confined time. I got a sense of what her world is like."

Remember that sensitivity to timing can pertain to clock time, calendar time, or biological time. "She's more hyper, impatient, and moody before her period," Heidi's mother said.

Teenagers change rapidly, so don't expect a talk in the car or some other such opportunity to be a sure thing tomorrow. "What I find with my kid is that you never know," Michael's mother said. "Every day is different. On an upbeat day you can talk to him about anything. The next day he could be down, and then he's like a pit bull."

As a cotherapist, you're going to have to make big adjustments to get your depressed teenager talking. His energy cycle may clash with yours. While you may be eager to talk in the bright light of morning, your teenager may be groggy and silent—or sleeping. Many teenagers come alive at night when the house is quiet and the distractions fewer. He may be ready to open up when you're ready to turn in. Steel yourself for late-night talks if you want to keep the communication lines open.

2. Create opportunities for privacy. Although it's nice to have the family gather at dinner, this is not a good forum for deep conversations with a depressed teen. The dinner table ought to be reserved for family members to exchange their news of the day, and it is too public for the kind of conversation you need to have. "The best time to talk is when no one else is around," Jennie's mother said. "We'll go on dates, just the two of us. Shopping often does it, although it's a sacrifice for me because I hate shopping."

I found that "coffee conversations" with Eric were productive. I'd take him out to a coffee bar, a private but "cool" venue for a conversation. Like most teenage boys, Eric was not one for lengthy discussions. The coffee provided a built-in timer, so that Eric didn't feel he'd be trapped into talking too long. When the coffee was finished, so were we.

3. Don't overstay your welcome. You have a limited amount of time during which you can keep a teen engaged in a conversation about a subject as sensitive as emotional health. The boys are worse than the girls. "I would go up to his room and sit on his bed," Jared's mother said. "If the TV was on, I wouldn't necessarily turn it off. I had fifteen to twenty minutes max before his eyes started glazing over." It's better to have frequent short conversations than one long, unproductive one. This can be exasperating when you want to finish a discussion. But you may have to settle for stop-and-start conversations rather than closure.

4. Keep track of every detail. "He gives me little parcels of information at inopportune times because he is embarrassed or guilty," Jason's mother said. "Once he told me, 'Mom, I got Brianna pregnant.' Then he rushed off. I would have to go back and tell him he left me with some pretty loaded stuff. It took me a year to put all the details together on what happened with that pregnancy. I kept listening, and I eventually got it all."

5. Be authentic. If you look as if you're merely going through the motions, you can't accomplish anything. "Authenticity is the number one prerequisite," Jared's mother said. "I'm up-front with him. I'm genuine. I don't disguise my true feelings. For instance, if I don't like his behavior, I tell him. Kids love the truth. Kids really want someone to listen. I make eye contact and stay focused on his face. I truly listen. It makes the relationship authentic. That's how kids will talk forever."

6. *Make an agenda.* Teenage depression seems to involve a central issue. For Jared, it was "the nemesis of the day," his mother said. "Wherever he is, he always tries to find a bad guy. He would feel victimized and then pick out the people he thought responsible. Then he would dwell on them and talk about them constantly."

For Carla, the central issue was relationships. For Michelle, it was conforming to rules. For Eric, it was self-esteem. However, identifying the central issue doesn't make it simple for you, because it has many subissues. I needed to make checklists for Eric to make sure I covered all aspects as they displayed themselves, and there were many. Moreover, Eric was still too young to tell me how to rank the items in order of importance. The item that got second billing on Tuesday might actually be the crux of his depression. I watched my list and covered all aspects. I couldn't afford to miss.

7. *Remember that teens are not sophisticated thinkers.* You must put things in simple terms. Moreover, you may have to head for the same destination the next day—but by traveling a different route. For the time being, settle for a good result even if you believe that the course in getting there was wrong. Their map may be written in a language you don't understand.

It helps to relate your point directly to the teenager's experience. Eric told me he went into the lunchroom and found it hard to find someone to sit with. Instead of a general statement about what a wonderful, likable guy he was, I gave him a specific rebuttal to consider: "Then why did your classmates elect you vice president of the sophomore class?" And, "Why did thirty kids want to come to a party at your house and hang out in your room?" As evidence, I showed him a photo of thirty friends happily crammed into his room.

8. *Adopt their feelings.* You can't explain their behavior or convince them to change if you come at them from your point of view. "Everything is friends," Carla's mother said. "It's a large issue. All three of her suicide attempts were over boyfriends. She's focusing her life on them. When a friend has upset her, I cannot get through to her. I don't even try." You may not like it at all, but you will have to become good at seeing things the way they do and explaining their feelings to their teachers.

Even when a teenager's concerns seem shallow, you have to give them some attention. Consider the cataclysmic impact of a "Rudolph"—a pimple blooming on the end of a teenager's nose. To you it might seem like a ridiculous thing to get worked up about, but to a teenager it can be the mark of Cain.

9. *Remember that direction is more important than magnitude.* I had to be patient with Eric. His ability to ultimately understand that every rejection or perceived snub was not intended personally took several years. During that long, slow process, while his self-esteem took a daily pounding, I had to be content with a little bit of progress here and there. I'm pleased he has arrived, but it was frustrating and painful to watch for so long a time.

10. *Be a detective.* It's not always enough to get a teenager talking—you have to determine if she's saying enough and telling the truth. "You have to be a loving interrogator," Alison's stepfather said. "Kids put up terrific ground cover. They hide well. Sometimes Alison would pretend to have a meaningful conversation, but it was just to get the damned thing over with."

Teenagers lie well, too, and the lies may be significant when the teen is depressed. As a cotherapist you must listen carefully and assess the truthfulness of what your teenager tells you.

11. *Stick to your guns.* Your teen may refuse to talk on certain occasions and try to ignore you or shout you down. "That's when I would have a 'hard talk' with Jared," his mother said. "I would tell him, 'I have the right and responsibility as a parent to say this.' There was no beating around the bush. I would quickly tell him exactly how I saw things. It was a fifty-fifty chance. Sometimes he didn't respond." A different kind of challenge comes from an ex-spouse giving your teen contradictory opinions. If you believe you are right, don't be afraid to hold your ground.

Ten Don'ts for Talking to Your Teen

1. Don't mandate. "With Michelle, I never tried to legislate new ways of thinking," her father said. "It would have been impossible because of her opposition to us." Moreover, mandating a change doesn't give the teen ownership of the change, and some teens won't believe that any rule for change will work unless it comes from within them. Inspire instead. And if all you can inspire in the beginning is just a change in behavior without the important change in attitude, it's okay. The attitude change may come later. It did with Eric.

2. Never do verbal battle. "I shouted at him and gave him an ultimatum," Jason's mother said. "I said, 'Quit the slug life, and I'm going to give you a deadline.' He's six-one and a one-hundred-and-seventy-five-pounder. He came at me, in the same spot in the kitchen just like his father did when Jason was seven." A physical altercation was averted, but Jason's mother learned the hard lesson that nothing can be accomplished through a verbal battle with a teenager. If the discussion degenerates into a screaming match, walk away. Come back to it tomorrow.

3. Avoid the word "wrong." I can't think of a quicker way to shut down a conversation. When the W-word gets blurted out, the teen goes from listening to saving face. No one listens well when they're on the defensive, especially someone as fragile as a depressed teen.

"I never told Michelle she was wrong even when it was obvious to both of us," her father said. "Instead, I would say, 'Let's try this another way,' or, 'Maybe this will work better.'"

4. Don't make personal judgments. It's tempting and easy, for example, to ascribe a person's negative thinking to laziness. Remember that depression is a disease, not a weakness or character flaw. You must speak to your teen just as a doctor speaks to an obese person about weight control—the doctor distinguishes the person from the weight problem. Similarly, try to reassure your teenager that the qualities that need changing are the qualities of the depression, not the qualities of bad behavior. After all, a doctor wouldn't accuse a teenager of being diabetic because he purposely sabotaged his own pancreas's insulin production.

5. Don't dwell on unimportant details. Specifically, these are the details that annoy parents. Jared's mother said it this way: "Don't major in the minors. I talk to a lot of teens as part of my church activities. Once I had a kid called Spike in my front seat. He put his right foot on the dash and against the windshield. I didn't say anything. He said, 'You're so cool. My mom would have gone ballistic.'"

6. Don't forget the humor. It breaks down barriers. At times Eric would be so steeped in depression he couldn't get out of bed. Instead of becoming angry, I would grab some percussion instruments like the maracas and tambourine we kept by the piano, go into his bedroom, and turn myself into a smiling one-man percussion band. I was a loud and annoying alarm clock. He would smile back and joke that next to the word *obnoxious* in the dictionary is my picture. Hostilities averted, we would both laugh and then talk a bit about what the day might confront him with.

7. Don't run on empty. Nearly every parent I interviewed has used the words *exhausted* or *overwhelmed* when they describe parenting a depressed teen. Face it. You'll have to look for some spare energy. A conversation when you're fatigued comes off as lifeless or insincere. Maybe it will never occur at all. You have only a certain amount of time and energy. If you're running on empty, pick a better time to talk. If you're always on empty, see how you might adjust your schedule. Economic realities may interfere, but do what you can. Jason's mother looks back this way: "I was working full-time. I should have worked half-time. They say they need you less when actually they need you more."

8. Don't retreat because of your own vulnerability. The more of yourself you put into a conversation, the more vulnerable you are. Because you are recommending some values, you are an easier target. You stand out more when you take a stand. You might hear, "How can you say that when you don't follow that advice yourself?" Or, "How can you help me when you've screwed up your own life so bad?" But you can turn your perceived vulnerability into an asset. Jared's mother did. "I never felt vulnerable," she said, "because I used my past rebellious experiences as examples. When the time was right during our talks, I would tell him about them."

9. Don't promise something that is undeliverable. You lose all credibility and trust.

10. Don't criticize your ex-spouse. "You can't say things about an ex-parent," Dan's mother said, "unless you want to set your kid against you. It's best to leave it for the context of a therapist or pastor, who can get rid of the emotions. At their age and emotional level, they're not ready. They can criticize, but you can't."

Fractured Communication

If you have a good relationship with your teen, you will usually be able to engage her in conversation and, perhaps, even inspire change. Sadly, some parent-teen relationships will never be good. Or, some relationships go through a troubled time during which communication breaks down for too long. What to do then?

Jenni's mother speaks from her experience as a teacher of highly resistant teenagers, many of whom have been in trouble with the law. "When a teenager is angry, step away from it until the situation calms," she said. "Nothing good will come of a screaming match with a child. It's not something you want to win. Directly after they have an outbreak is the time to talk. [It's] the calm after the storm. They are spent. They don't have the ability to fight and argue. And they want to reopen the lines of communication."

Fractured communication is the saddest of all possible situations for a parent. The opportunity to be a guide and helper is lost. The teen's pain continues unabated. Hope wanes. Carla's mother faced an especially difficult situation: "She'll lock herself in her room. I'll ask her to come out and visit, but she won't. She'll start sobbing in there and refuse to talk. When she gets upset with me, she'll lash out. She even struck me once." Selling advice to someone who won't listen is useless.

All this is not a showstopper. Carla's mother was wise enough to recruit mentors for Carla. "She has an aunt she will talk to—because she does it in a goofy way to get her to laugh. She talked to a youth director at our church a couple of times. This one knocks me over. Carla tried to jump off the [highway] 101 bridge twice. The second time a lady who lives down the road from here stopped her from jumping. You know, Carla's kept in touch with her, and they talk." Teens crave adult conversations to help clear up the fog that adolescence and depression confront them with every day. If you're not allowed to provide that conversation, find someone whom they will welcome. The stakes are too high to do otherwise.

Fractured communication doesn't mean you are now a nonparticipant in your teen's recovery. Even when you can't talk, you can communicate through example. "This was the tactic I used," said

Michelle's father. "I made sure my wife and I always showed by example that we were positive and optimistic about ourselves—and especially about her." So important is the notion of example that many moral theologians have devoted their lives to its study. For some, example is considered such a powerful influence that a moral transgression committed in "public" ought to be doubled in its wrongfulness because it gives a bad example. I don't doubt for an instant that my wife and I have influenced Eric more with our example than with any clever words.

Finally, you can communicate with your teenager through the written word. It's a wired age, and for teens e-mails are especially effective. Make them short and to the point. Your teen might even read a few of them. Even if this isn't a last resort, it's good practice anyway. If your teen goes away to college, you won't have the luxury of frequent face-to-face conversation. Start writing pointed and useful e-mails. You might as well learn to communicate with him the way the rest of his friends are doing right now.

Cognitive Features of Depression

Once you've overcome the barriers to communication, you can start to practice the subtle skills of a parent cotherapist. Besides patience and determination, you need a basic understanding of the cognitive aspects of depression.

Your perspective on life makes an extraordinary difference in your emotional health. Your perspective will largely determine whether an event in life is stressful, and then how you deal with the stress. Time and again researchers have shown that if your perspective doesn't jibe with reality, then you are a set up for depression and anxiety syndromes.

For example, one notable study showed that children who are depressed view themselves as less capable than nondepressed children even though their teachers viewed both groups as equally clever. Distorted and negative thinking about their self-evaluations got these children into trouble with their mental health. In fact, abnormal cognition is such a frequently observed characteristic of depression that it is considered a central feature of the illness. Depressed teens themselves will admit that their thinking is more negative than that of their friends or family, and that their thinking is more negative when they are depressed than when they are not.

Eric can force a laugh now about his distorted thinking in high school, but it caused intense distress when he was a sophomore. For example, he had quite a crush on Liz, a tenth-grade classmate: "She was prime. I tried to make her laugh, and she never seemed to laugh as much as I thought she should. I would always say hi, but she never talked to me in a way that made me happy. I thought I was a reject." It all came clear about a year later when Liz approached Eric and admitted the same kind of distorted thinking. "I was afraid to talk to you," she said. You were Eric Berlinger, and you were on the student council. You always had people around you." That sophomore year, Eric's self-evaluations tormented him because they almost always came out strongly negative. So did his evaluations of events in which he was a participant. "I couldn't see people for how they were really reacting. It was like I was looking at them through a sheet of waxed paper. All I could go on was what my head said. Depression made high school a nightmare." Eric's self-esteem notched down every time he took stock of himself. He sorely needed a prescription for healthy thinking.

Rx for Healthy Thinking

Johnny Mercer and Harold Arlen offered their own prescription in *Here Come the Waves,* a World War II movie released by Paramount pictures on New Year's Day, 1944. But they didn't get it completely right. In that movie, Bing Crosby played a crooner staging musical revues intended to recruit women into the armed forces. He belted out Mercer and Arlen's new song "Ac-cent-tchu-ate the Positive," making it an instant classic. The lyrics were intended to be the songwriters' formula for healthy thinking during some of the dark and depressing days of that horrific war, and it earned them an Oscar nomination.

Psychologists and psychiatrists would agree that we need to accentuate the positive for mental health. Depression, they say, is clearly related to a deficiency of positive thinking. Moreover, you need loads of positive thinking since studies show that it has less potency than negative thinking. At first glance, then, it would seem that Mercer and Arlen may have been right on the mark. If you accentuate positive thinking and eliminate negative thinking, you create ideal conditions to foster optimal mental health.

However, it only works that way in song. If you follow the rest of their prescription and "eliminate the negative," the result is giddiness, euphoria, narcissism, and even mania. Eliminating all the negatives eliminates contact with reality. Being out of touch with reality is definitely not emotional health. The genuine prescription for healthy thinking is not to delete every negative, but only those that are incorrect, unrealistic, or derived from faulty reasoning. Maintaining authentic negatives, and not sending them to the mind's recycle bin, yields precision thinking. Precision is what healthy thinking is all about.

Moreover, healthy thinking means the balance is shifted toward the positive. In fact, psychologists who call themselves cognitive-behavioral therapists have actually performed experiments to figure out mathematical formulas for what balance entails. After all, as Lord Kelvin is reputed as having said, "When you can say something with numbers, then you really know what you are talking about." Although it is an oversimplification of the formulas, this is what they have discovered: As long as the thoughts are accurate, the perfect balance for mental health is characterized by about two positive thoughts for each negative thought. Depression occurs when the ratio becomes one to one or worse. And, yes, more than two positive thoughts for each negative one means you are overly optimistic and verging on mania or some other mental affliction characterized by a wholly unjustified feeling of well-being.

And now, the caveat about precision.

All these formulas are mathematically correct on paper. But that's not quite the way they should get applied to real-life situations. The ratio of two positive thoughts to one negative thought actually requires a bit, just a bit, of imprecise thinking—but not in the negative direction. Emotionally healthy individuals possess positive views of themselves that are slightly unrealistic. They have a slightly exaggerated belief in their ability to control their circumstances. And they believe that their futures will turn out to be a bit better than the average person's. Remember Maria's words in *West Side Story* as she sang "I Feel Pretty" on a Spanish Harlem tenement roof. She felt pretty and witty enough to boast that perhaps "Miss America should just resign."

So here is what the prescription for mental health turns out to be in practice. Don't eliminate the genuine negatives. Make sure the positive thoughts tip the scales in the positive direction. And it's okay to overestimate the positive, to make it all slightly grand.

This is more than just a prescription for overall mental health. Cognitive-behavioral therapists believe it is likely a specific antidote for depression, and it may even prevent recurrences later in life. They say the depressed teen has a negative view of himself, a negative view of the world, and a negative view of the future. The scales tip wrongly because one side is loaded down with extreme pessimism, self-denigration, and self-blame.

Just remember the details of the prescription. You should not try to eliminate genuine negatives. If your teen is unattractive, argumentative, or impulsive, you can't deny the obvious. Instead, own up to it until you can implement a remedy, if there is one. Moreover, psychologists have considerable doubt that genuine negatives can ever completely be dislodged from one's memory anyway. Eric would agree that you waste valuable psychic energy trying to pretend some of those awful things never really happened that awful way. And make sure your teen "latches onto the affirmative." She should work to develop enough new positive qualities and new positive thoughts to tip the scales decisively. And remember, it takes about two positives to counteract one negative, so she—and you—have your work cut out for you.

Eric was especially challenging in this regard. He had gotten himself into a vicious circle. He considered himself unworthy of being anyone's friend. So he accommodated, but in self-defeating ways. He began to associate with the "dirtbags" of the school, as he called them, thinking he would be welcome among them. He took up dirtbag habits with them, like regularly chewing smokeless tobacco in the back of Miss Madison's advanced algebra class. Instead of learning mathematical terms during fifth period, he was learning the group's jargon of *chaw, chopper,* and *dip.* Thank goodness he didn't take up with the potheads or the goths. He became convinced that a second-rate person like himself belonged in second-rate groups, and he began to think like them—defeatist, negative, unambitious, and angry at the world for the raw deal. To complete the vicious circle, when he could muster the nerve to take a chance and make overtures to some of the nicer kids, he became instantly nervous and thought the best way to gain acceptance was to be humorous and entertaining. It's hard even for a professional to do stand-up comedy, and only the raconteur can sparkle with extemporaneous cool and clever conversation. Eric being neither, his valiant attempts would often fall flat, and he would estrange those he was trying to entertain. The repeated failures reinforced his sense of worthlessness, and he went back to the dirtbags.

That's a lot of bad thinking to undo, and that was only a small fraction of it. I started scanning Eric's remarks for clues like "I'm going to the football game by myself. Maybe I'll meet up with someone." I could discern when his self-talk was telling him to hide from people and he wasn't intending to meet anyone at all. I surveyed his behavior. For example, he wouldn't play a tennis match with the verve of his partner. Although talented, at times like that he was pessimistic about the match, the day, and the future.

I began making daily lists based on my observations of Eric. I wrote down things I had to speak to him about right away, things that shouldn't wait past tomorrow, and things that needed repeated discussion every week or so. I attended to every item. Sometimes all those lists seemed silly, and I would feel like an overprotective, intrusive, and neurotic parent. A few times that proved true, and I'm sure I appeared absurd. But not to continually intervene in this dreadful disease is even more absurd. So I persisted, even in the face of occasional defeat. When Eric didn't want to listen, he knew I valued him so much as to be dearly interested in him. When Eric couldn't listen, at least he knew I would be there as a safety net. And when Eric couldn't act on our conversation, he might still recall it later and put it to use then. He told me this only last year, and I am reassured by that revelation. But those times when I got through made me feel especially like his champion. When his thinking changed for the better, his depression lightened. He became more hopeful and felt more worthy, and he could start digging himself out of the hole. I asked him yesterday about his vicious circle, and he told me, "I don't think like that anymore." He said it with a bittersweet smile on his face, but it was still a smile.

Checklist for Cotherapy at Home

To be an effective cotherapist for your teen, focus on these goals.

Get rid of negative distortions. Dr. Aaron Beck was a pioneer psychologist who cataloged the cognitive distortions that afflict depressed people. These are the ones that seem especially important for teens. If you see any of them, put them on your list, and talk to your teen about them:

- Depressed teens focus on **negative details** in a situation and ignore or undervalue the positive ones or the more important ones. The conclusion gets twisted in the wrong direction. Eric always seemed to remember the negative details of an encounter with another person and usually painted the encounter as painful or embarrassing. He even seemed to remember the negative events depicted in a movie more than the positive ones.

- Depressed teens can come to **unjustified negative conclusions** in the absence of any negative evidence whatsoever.

- Depressed teens tend to think in **absolute terms.** There are only extremes, and no shades of gray. If I'm bad, I must be horrible. If I have acne, I must be ugly.

- **Overgeneralization** is particularly nefarious. If I failed at soccer, I will also fail at math, dance, and making friends. If one particular boy doesn't like me, all boys must dislike me. Certainly, then, my parents can't like me either.

- **Catastrophizing.** To think that the sky is falling is a laughable bad habit only if you're not depressed. However, when you are depressed, it makes life an eternal dread. Only the worst of all possible outcomes is seen as likely, and a negative life event, even a minor one, can have only severe negative life consequences. If I can't get a date this weekend, I will never be loved. I will never get married. I will be alone forever.

- **Taking things personally.** If they didn't invite me to the party, I know it's because I'm a geek. Eric was particularly adept at this thinking distortion. No, he wasn't a geek. Maybe the party was only for hockey jocks or kids from a certain neighborhood. Maybe it was only for kids whose parents schmoozed with each other.

Get rid of the negative mind-set. Depressed teens pepper their speech with more negative adjectives than positive ones. They recall more negative events than positive events, and they can come to a negative conclusion faster than a positive one. You must point this out, because depressed teens usually are unaware of their thinking patterns. With your help, they might be able to convince themselves that they are in a negative rut and might then start weighing evidence.

Get rid of automatic thoughts. Depressed teens may come to a conclusion before they have carefully thought it over. Automatically, they decide on the negative, the gloom, the self-denigration. "My life is a total mess" might be the most common negative automatic thought for a depressed teen. Whenever anything bad or untoward happens, this thought immediately comes to mind. It explains the bad occurrence and predicts the inevitable future futility. But who said her life is a total mess? Where did that idea come from? Can she prove it? Who is keeping that tally?

Get rid of rumination. This is one of the worst habits depressed teens get stuck in. Eric would stay awake until the small hours of the morning going over his supposed failings again and again. When he could drag himself out of bed for school, he would go over the same material while he was in the shower. On the drive to school, he would repeat it a third time. Stop! If only it were as easy as running around the block a few times to get out of it. Different tricks work for different people. Determine what technique for immediate distraction works for your teen. Maybe it's singing a song. Maybe it's setting to work on a physically demanding task. By trial and error, you should be able to discover what works for your teen. Breaking the rumination cycle will require your help.

Get rid of the defective attributional style. If I failed, it's purely my fault, because I screw up everything I try. In addition, whatever is in me won't ever change or go away. If I succeeded, certainly it was only because a particular person was helping me with that particular task. Or maybe I was just lucky this time. This is how a depressed teenager with defective attributional style thinks.

Recently, Eric got himself a research internship in a leading medical center. "I did it myself," he was pleased to announce. "You didn't do it for me this time." A couple of years ago, he would have assumed that I had greased the skids for him even if I hadn't. He wouldn't have allowed himself to feel that sense of accomplishment.

Tailor your emphasis. Dr. Beck categorized depressed people according to the importance they place on social interactions. The "sociotropic" person emphasizes social relationships. Failures here are kindling and matchsticks for depression, because this kind of teen places a premium on affection and acceptance. If this description fits your teen, much of your talk should focus on friendships. Your teen is not being frivolous—this is where he derives much of his comfort and gratification. Beck's other category is "autonomous." These people derive satisfaction and their sense of worth from accomplishing meaningful tasks and acting independently. If this describes your child, failures at schoolwork or with personal projects will be his focus, and your talk will need this kind of emphasis.

Teach social skills. Teens are just beginning to develop a repertoire of social skills. Their skills are not fine-tuned, and many teens turn out to be just plain clumsy in social settings. This is a disaster for a depressed teen, because a good social performance yields positive reinforcement, boosting one's self-concept. That can counteract depression. A bad performance exacerbates depression. Which skills to emphasize depends on the teen. Some teens need to learn how to engage in conversation. Others have difficulty recognizing another's emotions, and that is a huge impediment to successful interpersonal interactions. Still, others need to learn how to give negative feedback in a constructive manner to another person, and to make sure that positive feedback never gets omitted when deserved. Finally, due to depression's inherent anger and irritability, some teens will need coaching on how to solve social conflicts. A conversation may be sufficient, or you may have to do a bit of role-playing with your teen. Teens who suffer comorbidity with ADHD or any of the anxiety syndromes may have especially deficient skills and often need the help of a professional.

Teach self-control. I can't think of a single talent that is more important in the fight against depression. Simply put, self-control gives us mastery over our impulses. Eric needed self-control over his negative automatic thoughts. He would awaken each morning and automatically say, "Oh, shit," at the realization another day had started, and he was dark from the get-go. He had to discipline himself into awakening with a different attitude, and it didn't have to be overwhelmingly positive to be effective.

Failure to gain mastery over a bad trait may be generalized as incompetence for all traits. The result is helplessness. When depression bestows hopelessness, the combination can be deadly. Fortunately, the opposite is also true. Teens will use the ability to control one aspect of the day as proof that they can indeed control other aspects, and self-control burgeons with each achievement.

11

Strategy Nine
Look beyond Therapy

I was wrong.

When I first heard the story as a young medical student, I assumed it was factual. It was supposed to have happened at my own medical school, the University of Michigan, sometime just before I started there. As the story goes, a professor was taking medical students on early-morning rounds through the pediatric cancer ward. The professor stopped at a certain bedside, and to check on whether the students had studied the charts of the young people hospitalized there, he asked the group, "What do we have here?" No one knew the diagnosis. "A Wilms' tumor," the professor said. To correct what was perceived as an unacceptable view of illness, one of the medical students impudently interjected, "You must mean a Wilms' tumor—and with a patient attached." I told that satisfying story a few times to family and friends to illustrate that a doctor must never forget a fundamental tenet of medicine—a disease in one corner of the body can affect the entire body. I also bragged that my medical school was so enlightened that its students and professors heartily subscribed to that idea. About twenty years later, one of my medical colleagues told me a virtually identical story—and how it had happened at his own medical school. He bragged, too. The story turned out to be apocrypha.

As a medical student, I was delighted to have found myself training among people who were concerned about caring for the entire patient. I will always remember many of my classmates' answers about why they wanted to become doctors. Seldom did they say they wanted to stamp out a particular disease or learn how to operate on colons or knees. More often, their primary orientation was the whole patient rather than just the disease. The most stirring response, and I am sorry I've forgotten who said it, was "I want to take care of the folks." In that person's mind, there were always people attached to their afflictions.

As I look back on my medical school years, the sixties were indeed a decade of huge technological advances in medicine. Also, the results of a new breed of rigidly conceived and well-performed scientific studies were pouring in to establish the venerable yardstick of evidence-based medicine. Anecdote was finally being discarded in favor of scientific inquiry. The triumph was that old-time diseases with descriptive names like *consumption, dropsy,* or *ague* were being discarded for more precise formulations like *tuberculosis, ascites,* or *malaria.* As diseases were being discovered to originate in certain compartments of the body, however, the danger was approaching that the compartment, rather than the whole patient, would command the physician's attention. Doctors weren't forgetting there was a patient attached, but it was getting harder to remember.

Henry Emmons, M.D., always remembers. He is a Twin Cities

psychiatrist who has been requested by six local colleges and universities to care for their depressed students. He received his psychiatric training at the University of Rochester and is an adjunct professor at the University of Minnesota Medical School's renowned Center for Spirituality and Healing.

"I think depression is a premier example of a whole-body disease," Dr. Emmons said. "It's not just the brain that's involved. It's the endocrine system, too, because that system produces the stress hormones involved in the way the disease unfolds. The gut is also involved, because the intestines are rich in serotonin. Depression manifests itself in many places in the body. It's not only the brain's thinking that doesn't go right and gets out of control. You see a depletion of energy, sex drive, and appetite. Diurnal rhythms get altered, too. I never want parents to shy away from [antidepressant] medicines when they're needed. But these medicines treat only the brain. They just manipulate the metabolism of serotonin. My belief is that with these medicines the other underlying causes aren't addressed. Medicines don't treat the entire patient."

The entire patient is not just the entire protoplasmic body. The concept of the entire patient also includes the cultural and societal milieu. Karen Dawson, M.D., heartily supports this view. She is a family practitioner who treats many depressed adolescents, especially young girls with comorbid eating disorders. She is also the current president of the American Holistic Medical Association. I asked her to explain her views.

Q. *How do you, as a holistic doctor, view adolescent depression?*

A. It is more complicated than just a genetic predisposition or a low serotonin level. I must examine how that person is contained in her culture or society. For instance, there are epidemics of depression that are unique to our Western culture. If I don't look at the big picture, I am going to be missing many important factors. I have to back up and do what my dad used to recommend—take the thirty-thousand-foot view.

Q. *How do you define your kind of practice?*

A. I define it as a focus on the whole person. I also include remembering that some complementary or alternative therapies may be helpful with certain patients. Basically, I try to appreciate the uniqueness of each patient. I want to understand all aspects of their emotional, societal, and spiritual health. I think it is critical to model hope and optimism to them. I essentially tell them that I don't see the depression in front of me. I see the hope, even if she can't see it.

Q. *Please give a few examples of the other kinds of things you do for a depressed teen besides prescribing antidepressants.*

A. The best thing I can do is give people skills for reflection and self-exploration. I also try to give them skills to cope with the stressors of life, whether it is the darkness of winter or the stressor of an exam. I insist that they cultivate a daily practice in a quiet time to observe who they are. This could be prayer, controlled breathing, meditation, or some kind of relaxation. Then they will be able to say to themselves, "When I am in this painful place, there is still a core of me that is healthy." I also ask them to keep a journal. When teens get really depressed, they lose contact. They should write their insights down so they can remember them.

Q. *Do you think a parent should view their child's depression the same way?*

A. It's intuitive for most people that depression is a multifactorial disease. You cannot separate an adolescent's depression from her worldview. Parents should try to understand how the symptoms of depression fit into the whole of her life. They should ask what her passion in life is. They have to ask what her beliefs are. The kind of belief system she has will determine what kinds of symptoms she has with her depression.

Q. *How actively do you involve parents in the treatment of their teen's depression?*

A. Parents can provide on a daily basis what I provide only on a weekly basis. If the parents aren't ill themselves, they must be harnessed as a resource. It is critical. I ask the teen's permission, and then I start the conversation between her and her parents right away. It needs to be done delicately, though, because there may be anger issues on both sides. Parents are incredibly tuned in to the "extra" things that need to be done. There is nothing more effective than a motivated parent.

I asked Dr. Emmons and Dr. Dawson to help me compile a list of specific things a depressed teen should do to fight back besides antidepressants and psychotherapy. The parents I interviewed added their own suggestions, too. I am a scientist by training, and I reminded all of them that I believe wholeheartedly in evidence-based medicine. The things all these people told me had to make good scientific sense. Better yet, their recommendations should have some endorsement by scientific experimentation. Here is the essence of our conversations.

Exercise: The Natural Antidepressant

In 1998, the National Center for Health Statistics published a landmark study. Statisticians had carefully surveyed over fifty-five thousand people in the United States and Canada to determine whether physical activity promotes mental health. The conclusion was inescapable. Physical activity promotes a positive mood and a sense of general well-being. It also decreases the symptoms of anxiety and depression. Moreover, the relationship held up for both genders and all age groups, and it was independent of socioeconomic status. Exercise, it seemed, helped everyone. A vast scientific literature has accumulated since then, all of it in agreement.

If exercise maintains mental health, the obvious question a doctor would ask next is whether it can effectively treat emotional illness, especially depression. This literature is not so vast, but the results are striking. For mild or moderate depression, at least one study has documented that regular physical exercise is as good at reducing symptoms of depression as are antidepressant medications. There is no agreement, though, about how exercise works its beneficial effect. Some investigators point to a biochemical effect in the brain whereby levels of neurotransmitters or endorphins, the body's own feel-good molecules, are shifted in a favorable direction. Other scientists think that the mechanism is largely psychological: regular exercise increases feelings of self-efficacy, improves one's self-image, and diverts the mind from negative thoughts. The social contact it provides is likely an important mechanism for the teen who is especially withdrawn or isolated.

What is the exact prescription for exercise to get the best results in depression? Although there is no agreement, it seems not to matter. Scientists have studied all sorts of exercise—swimming, circuit training, jogging, aerobic dance, step aerobics, and tae kwon do, to name just a few. Any of them reduces anger, confusion, fatigue, and symptoms of depression and anxiety. Scientists are getting even more enthusiastic about exercise as a "drug" to combat depression, because further studies have shown it doesn't matter if it is aerobic or nonaerobic, low-intensity or high-intensity, solitary or communal. It only needs to be frequent and regular. Exercise physiologists recommend that the exercise last at least forty minutes, be done three to six times a week, and continue for at least sixteen weeks.

Motivation is the biggest problem. How can you get your teen to exercise or play a sport when tackling the less strenuous or demanding tasks of daily living is a daunting challenge? That was the case with Eric. He was a talented member of his high school tennis team, but showing up for practices was a chore. I could no longer merely nag him from the stands. I had to get more actively involved. I had never played a single game of tennis before, but under the circumstances, I decided to take up the sport myself to become Eric's tennis "buddy" whether he wanted one or not. At middle age, trying a new sport could turn out to be a fool's errand. In many ways, it turned out worse. I would ask Eric to go "hit balls" outside on a nice summer's day, or indoors at a local tennis club on a cloudy winter weekend. On one of his angry days, he would either slam the ball back at me so that I could never get it, or he would try to "win the point" even though we were just trying to hit the ball back and forth as many times as possible. I enrolled us as a team in father-son tournaments, sometimes embarrassing him because I seldom achieved even mediocrity. Often, he considered his father-partner more of a challenge than the opponents on the other side of the net. I even sprained an ankle trying to improve my skills "on the sly" during a beginner's drill. My tennis career lasted a couple of years. Fearing more injuries and more humiliation, I happily gave it up when Eric's depression remitted. Still, I saw the proof of the scientific studies in front of me: I saw that Eric almost always came off the court less depressed than he went on it, even if I had to drag him there—and even if he had to play with me. It was well worth it.

Meditation: Keep a Clear Mind

Mention meditation to some people and they immediately turn up their noses. They think meditation always comes with the trappings of mysticism, spiritual goals, unfamiliar cultural practices, religious beliefs, or bearded gurus. Sometimes this is so, but that is not what I am talking about here. Meditation can be stripped of all these trappings and still retain its identity and full force as a healthy practice. Furthermore, meditation does not mean "zoning out" by making the mind go blank or stopping thought processes. On the contrary, meditation only clears the mind of its distracting noises—sadness, anger, worry, doubt. As a result, the mind becomes more active, but in decidedly constructive ways. Meditation can be defined as "the voluntary deployment of attention." To meditate, one doesn't need chants, tapes, incense, a sunset, or a spa. It can be done anytime one can take a break from the din and bustle of daily living. One needs only to concentrate.

"There are two major branches of meditation," Dr. Emmons said. "One is focus meditation. You use something like a mantra, rosary beads, a scriptural passage, or a centering prayer. You use it to settle the mind down so that you can contact a place of spiritual quiet. The other type is mindfulness meditation. It's used in hundreds of hospitals and clinics throughout the country."

Mindfulness meditation requires that a person become acutely aware of all circumstances of the present moment. While you are reading this book, for example, mindfulness meditation requires that you look at the color of the paper, feel its texture, appreciate how your body feels sitting in the chair, take notice of what position your hands and feet are in, consider the direction and brightness of the lighting, and so on. On top of that, you must become "nonjudgmental." That means you must not in any way evaluate the experience of reading this page. The result will be total immersion in this moment.

That should automatically rid the brain of its own noise. Noise-free, the mind becomes tranquil, and that allows a person a few moments to think clearly.

"With either method of meditation the end results are the same," Dr. Emmons said. "One benefit is that you get a calming of the mind. I think that both anxiety and depression are signs of a mind gone rampant. Another benefit is that you can focus your thinking. You can question the validity of your thoughts, and you must do this constantly. Ancient wisdom says that what your mind dwells on is what grows for you. For example, if a relationship fails and you believe it was your fault, by dwelling on it, it will definitely become your fault whether it was or not. The way out of this is to question your thoughts. You get a front-row seat to your emotions and see them for what they are. Timing is really important. I don't think a depressed person can learn how to meditate while deeply depressed. They usually have to wait until the depression is pretty much over. Adolescence is an appropriate time to take it up." Already, studies show that scores on depression inventories improve with meditation.

"It's also very important to pursue meditation, because I think good meditation skills can prevent recurrences of depression," Dr. Emmons said. Since thoughts trigger moods, meditation seems to have a big theoretical advantage in preventing recurrences. It is important for a formerly depressed teen to distinguish whether today's thoughts are mere mental events or actual reflections of reality. The noise-stripping aspect of meditation may allow an accurate distinction rather than the furtherance of depressogenic thinking errors that may trigger another mood disturbance. Meditation allows a formerly depressed teen to come face-to-face with the validity of her emotions and interrupt the irrational thoughts before they get out of control. Recently, several randomized, controlled trials of combining mindfulness meditation with cognitive-behavioral therapy have shown sizable decreases in the recurrence rates of depression.

Yoga: Keep an Open Mind

There are enough similarities with meditation that yoga may be more than just a path toward general fitness. It might actually be a prescription for some of the medical problems that ail us. The National Institutes of Health agrees that yoga is worth a look. It has recently funded studies of whether a yoga regimen may benefit patients with multiple sclerosis. Its enthusiasm comes from past studies that showed that asthmatic patients who practiced yoga needed less asthma medication, and that patients with cardiovascular disease achieved increased cardiac endurance.

There is little scientific evidence, though, that speaks to the role of yoga in treating emotional illness. It is known that adherence to a regular yoga regimen significantly improves the course of obsessive-compulsive disorder. And scientific investigations have shown that yoga can improve a person's mood as much as vigorous swimming. Consequently, several studies of yoga's potential benefits for depressed patients have just been launched. Once they are published, you should be able to examine the results by logging on to PubMed. I wouldn't be surprised if yoga turned out to be somewhat helpful. Your depressed teen shouldn't necessarily rush out and look for a yoga instructor just yet, because the benefit may not go beyond the relaxation it provides. Still, if your teen has a comorbid anxiety disorder that denies him the ability to relax, yoga may be an important adjunct.

Diet and Dietary Supplements

In countries whose diets contain a low level of fish, the prevalence of depression seems to be high. Scientific investigators carried this observation further and found that depressed people have lower blood levels of omega-3 fatty acids, substances found usually in fish oils. Only one study, however, has been performed to determine whether fish oils can counteract depression. This study of bipolar patients came out positive, but studies of typical depression need to be done yet. Dr. Emmons is convinced right now, though, and he believes you needn't wait for these studies. "A teen's lunch and supper ought to include a frequent fish course, especially fatty fish such as salmon, herring, mackerel, or sardines," Dr. Emmons said. "These kinds of fish are rich in omega-3 fatty acids."

Neuropsychiatrists believe depression results from a deficiency in the brain's serotonin level. "Serotonin cannot be eaten in the diet," Dr. Emmons said. "The reason is that it gets degraded in the gut rather than absorbed into the blood. Serotonin must be manufactured by the body, and the building block is an essential amino acid called tryptophan. A teen's breakfast is either nonexistent or nothing more than a carbohydrate snack caught on the fly. This kind of breakfast is poor in tryptophan. This meal ought to have high-quality protein in it to provide a lot of tryptophan, things such as eggs, yogurt, or a protein powder. Don't forget the quality of the other meals, either."

In the eighties, capsules of chemically purified tryptophan were all the rage. Tryptophan was available at health food stores and widely used for depression. Unfortunately, its use resulted in a disease called eosinophilia-myalgia syndrome. This was not due to the tryptophan itself, but rather to a chemical contaminant introduced during its manufacture. As a consequence, in 1989 the FDA recalled all tryptophan-containing nutritional supplements in the United States, and they remain unavailable today. Nutritional scientists then shifted their attention to 5-hydroxytryptophan (5-HTP), a chemical intermediate on the way from tryptophan to serotonin. Several studies have concluded that 5-HTP is safe and shows definite promise against depression. But there's an important caveat: it causes side effects similar to SSRIs, and for this reason 5-HTP should not be taken concurrently with them.

The data for S-adenosylmethionine (SAM-e) are less clear, even though in Italy it outsells Prozac as an antidepressant. SAM-e is a brain chemical whose role in depression has yet to be made clear. Still, a number of scientific studies suggest that high blood levels of it may counter depression, although therapeutic and toxic doses need to be defined. SAM-e should not be taken concurrently with SSRIs.

Folate is a B vitamin that may have a large role in depression. Scientific studies show that up to one-third of depressed people have low folate levels, and the more depressed the folate level, the more severely depressed the person. Furthermore, a low folate level may predict a suboptimal response to a prescription antidepressant. Even though no randomized trial of folate in the treatment of depression has yet been conducted, it seems reasonable to ask your teen's doctor to consider a folate supplement. Don't overdo it, though. Ingestion of excessive quantities of folate pills may cause symptoms that actually mimic depression. "A teen's diet is usually not very high in green, leafy vegetables," Dr. Emmons said. "They're a good source of B vitamins. That's why I believe a depressed teenager should take a B-complex nutritional supplement that includes folate."

Herbs: Approach with Caution

Until several decades ago, about half of all prescription drugs were either derived from plants or were synthesized in pharmaceutical laboratories to have virtually the same chemical structures as the plant substances. For example, the best treatment for heart failure required use of a leaf extract of the digitalis plant or semisynthetic substances like it. During the Vietnam war, Chinese doctors became worried about how many of the participating Chinese troops were falling to malaria and began a search of plants for a quick and easy remedy. They happened upon artemisinin, a chemical constituent of the wormwood bush. Rigorous scientific investigations over the subsequent twenty years have proved its value against malaria so convincingly that the World Health Organization is contemplating its routine use, especially in poor countries where more expensive drugs seem to offer no advantage. Plant substances have remarkable healing powers, and many pharmaceutical and biotechnology companies are continuing the search for plant-derived substances like Taxol, the powerful anticancer drug derived from Pacific yew bark.

Many plants and herbs haven't fared as well. Ginkgo biloba, extracted from the leaves of the maidenhair tree, is supposed to ward off memory loss and dementia. Scientific studies can't confirm those claims. Echinacea was supposed to prevent the common cold or make its symptoms less severe, but it comes up short. The evidence remains unclear for valerian as a treatment for insomnia, and for saw palmetto to help the symptoms of an enlarged prostate. Perhaps the biggest failure is that of ginseng as a treatment for anything. Some herbs work. Some herbs don't.

Saint-John's-wort is the most commonly used antidepressant in Germany, and as many as 1 percent of adults in the United States have also used it for depression. Consequently, the National Institutes of Health's Center for Complementary and Alternative Medicine felt obliged to sponsor a large, well-controlled study to determine whether Saint-John's-wort was effective against depression according to stringent scientific criteria. The study, published in 2002, raised everybody's dander. It showed that Saint-John's-wort was no better than a sugar pill in treating depression of moderate severity. The critics of this herb felt justified in finally indicting it as a sham treatment and debunking the abundance of earlier studies suggesting it was effective. Proponents of the herb countered that the NIH study focused only on subjects who were quite severely depressed. Saint-John's-wort, they said, was intended to be used only for mild depression.

Although the debate rages on, several facts have come out in the wash. First, the NIH study clearly showed Saint-John's-wort was not of much use in moderate or severe depression. Until further scientific evidence is forthcoming, its use should probably be restricted to mild depression or seasonal depression popping up in the dark of winter. Second, Saint-John's-wort does indeed have side effects. This is unfortunate, since the main reason for choosing it over prescription antidepressants is to avoid troublesome side effects. In fact, Saint-John's-wort can cause gastrointestinal disturbances, difficulties achieving orgasm, dizziness, headache, frequent urination, or fatigue. Finally, Saint-John's-wort interferes with prescription drugs. It neutralizes the effects of indinavir, an anti-HIV drug, so much so that doctors are worried the combination of the two could result in resistance of the human immunodeficiency virus to indinavir, or to outright treatment failures. It also interferes enough with cyclosporine, an antirejection drug used in transplant recipients, so that a transplanted organ might even be rejected. There is a question whether it decreases the effect of birth control pills. If your teen is taking Saint-John's-wort, it is mandatory that her doctor be informed in order to avoid any potentially harmful drug interactions.

On top of this, many manufacturers of herbal remedies seem to have quality-control problems. The active ingredient in Saint-John's-wort is unknown. Even when manufacturers take a guess as to what it is, assays of that ingredient in capsules from different manufacturers show a variance of about 15 percent to a whopping 200 percent. Even assays of a single manufacturer's production may show a variance of over 150 percent from batch to batch. Worse yet, the plant may be contaminated with pesticides, animal waste, fumigants, or toxic metals. It is sadly ironic that anyone choosing an herb because it is "organic" may be exposed to unnatural and even dangerous contaminants. Finally, these manufacturers often have trouble designing something as simple as a pill or capsule that can release the herb at an appropriate time in the digestive tract. Various investigations have shown that some manufacturers' capsules don't liberate the herb until twenty hours after ingestion, when the capsule has usually already been excreted.

Depressed teens who have a comorbid anxiety disorder sometimes resort to kava for its calming effect. This effect appears to be real. In the eighteenth century, Captain Cook observed Polynesians using kava beverages as part of wedding celebrations or during ceremonies to welcome dignitaries. It induced a dreamy and desirable state of relaxation. Almost three hundred years later, it was easy to shop at a U.S. drugstore or supermarket and find shelves full of kava capsules, pills, extracts, or powders. Then, European reports of side effects began accumulating. People who ingested it were experiencing liver damage, sometimes so severe that a liver transplant was required to prevent death. Kava is now banned in Canada, Germany, and Singapore. The United States Food and Drug Administration (FDA) issued its own warning last year that kava is dangerous. The bottom line— don't allow your teen to use kava at all. Always check the label on any bottle of an herbal "mood enhancer" or "mood elevator" for its ingredients. I was recently surprised to leaf through the *Physicians' Desk Reference* (PDR) for the contents of various manufacturers' preparations of "pure" Saint-John's-wort. One of them listed kava among its numerous ingredients, despite the FDA warning.

The Importance of Sleep

When questioned, any neuroscientist who studies sleep will frankly admit that she doesn't know what purpose it really has. Moreover, little sleep research has ever been performed to determine exactly how, and how much, teens ought to sleep. Therefore, it's no surprise that there's no conclusion about what to do when a depressed teen shows disturbed sleep. Any disturbance is possible. The depressed teen may sleep too much, a condition called hypersomnia. More often, he has insomnia and sleeps too little. On top of too much or too little sleep, the sleep cycle may get reversed. The depressed teen may stay awake most of the night, then be sleepy or sleep during daylight. Eric experienced all three of these disturbances in a year. His sleeping became chaotic, and he became exhausted.

For the parent-partner it's important to remember what we do know about a teen's requirements for a good night's sleep, even though it's meager information. First, teens likely need about nine to ten hours of sleep each night, more than an average adult. Second, additional research shows that their sleep clock is shifted a bit. Compared to adults, they go to sleep later and get up later. Some school administrators have, in fact, become convinced that this is the normal state of affairs for teens and have changed high school start times from around 7:30 a.m. in their districts to around 8:30 a.m. Enlightened commanders at some military bases have delayed reveille an hour or two to accommodate the normal sleeping pattern and needs of the teenaged enlistees under their command.

Your first job will be to ensure that your depressed teen gets an appropriate amount of sleep. This is a difficult assignment for even an average teen, because a recent survey of high school freshman showed that 63 percent complain of daytime sleepiness owing to inadequate sleep. The average teen winds up with a late-night schedule because of jobs, socializing, sports, and homework, and teens say they want more sleep on weeknights. You can imagine how much worse the situation becomes for a depressed teen who has insomnia. Scientists have documented the consequences of too little sleep—decreased academic performance, significant behavioral difficulties,

difficulties with interpersonal relationships, and increased accidents. Depressed teens get a few others added to the list. Too little sleep seems to foster depression, it predicts illicit drug use and alcohol abuse as the insomniac teen "medicates" with these substances to achieve sleep, and it predisposes to suicide attempts. Maybe the worst aspect of insomnia, as it was for Eric, is too much time during the dark of night to venture into the dark corners of the troubled soul. Rumination over the day's failures and recalculation of self-worth, never coming out good, are principal activities for the depressed person awake in bed. With no one to talk to, the imagination takes over. The teen becomes afraid of the dark again.

Sleep problems are an aspect of depression that doctors often forget. Watch your teen's sleeping pattern carefully, because the morbidity of untreated insomnia is substantial. The correct first approach is the treatment of the underlying depression. The physician must try to prescribe antidepressant medicines that may have a side effect of drowsiness, here beneficial, that thus gets exploited in the evening. Insomnia can also clear with successful psychotherapy. If neither of these approaches seems to be succeeding, request that your teen's physician prescribe a separate sleep-inducing medicine such as a benzodiazepine.

Hypersomnia, sleeping too much, is the opiatelike oblivion that many depressed people seek as an escape. Unfortunately, too much sleep brings your depressed teen down even more, especially if the hypersomnia precludes being on time for school, participation in sports, or attendance at extracurricular activities. When that happens, self-esteem goes into an even steeper nosedive. It's better to rouse the seemingly unrousable, risk their anger as I did with Eric, and get them moving. As for many depressed people, Eric's depression was at its worst in the morning. To open his eyes and get out of bed was to awaken to a sentence of another intolerable day. But to stay in bed was worse. I used every trick possible. I would turn on the TV to CNN headline news and hope something might catch his interest and perhaps also distract him from his mood. I would sit on the edge of the bed and force him into a conversation. I would bring back a large cup of Caribou coffee, his favorite, and hope the aroma would force him to sit upright in bed and awaken a bit. I would fill his room with near-deafening noise, tell lame jokes, or pull the covers off his bed. I would laugh while doing it, and Eric had a good enough sense of humor that he could often laugh along. Usually it worked—and Eric realized he could wake up to something seemingly pleasant rather than to his own self-recriminations.

The Role of Spirituality

Religious involvement and spiritual beliefs almost unanimously get credit for a positive effect on mental health. Only one study I know of, though, has put this important notion to a scientific test. In a nationally representative sample of adolescent girls in grades seven through twelve, personal devotion and frequent participation in a religious community predicted a lower attack rate of depression. Moreover, the protection grows as teens get older and seems to last at least throughout the childbearing years. Modern mainstream psychotherapy has always accepted religious and spiritual issues as truly relevant to mental health.

Besides providing protection, religious and spiritual ideas also shape the way in which depressed people think about their emotional illness and respond to it. Scientists at Boston University surveyed depressed adults and found that religious and spiritual activities were their number one nonmedical "practice," more than yoga, herbs, or body-manipulation modalities such as massage. Moreover, these people claimed it promoted their recovery by increasing their sense of well-being, their "inner strength," and the ability to focus thoughts.

This finding was replicated for depressed teens by University of Nebraska scientists who found that those teens who participated more frequently in religious activities had lower scores on depression inventories. Scientifically speaking, religious and spiritual activities seem to decrease cognitive impairments. Spiritually speaking, these activities may mitigate the consequences of a terrible illness. Adolescence is a time of spiritual awakening. It would seem appropriate to encourage a depressed teen to go headlong into religious and spiritual discovery.

12

Strategy Ten
Consider Schools and Schedules

We all keep a mental list of treasured books that we consider unforgettable. They are the books we quote to friends. They are the ones we refer to for elucidation of some event or phenomenon. These books are unforgettable because they help define life experiences for us.

One on my list is *The Quest for Community* by Robert Nisbet. A premise of the book is that many Americans at home were in some ways saddened when World War II came to an end. The war had created a remarkable sense of community among those whose lives needed or wanted more of that sense. It was easy to talk to a stranger at a lunch counter or a bus stop about how combat in the Pacific theater was going. Mundane jobs were magically transformed into a communal "war effort." And the rationing of goods banded together otherwise nameless individuals who were now trying to find a way through or around that particular wartime hardship.

I am not old enough to remember any of World War II. After reading Nisbet's book, though, I had asked my father, who had received a draft notice in 1943, if any of Nisbet's contentions rang true. Yes, he said, quite a few. During the war years my father was a young man living in Detroit, the "Arsenal of Democracy." The book explained why, as a child in the fifties, I sometimes heard adults talking about "the war" with a peculiar nostalgia that I could not understand then. So, I am not surprised at the colossal popularity of recent movies about that war such as *Saving Private Ryan.* Neither am I mystified about why the History Channel has found a large and loyal viewership with its black-and-white programs about the planes, tanks, battles, and admirals of World War II. The grainy footage resurrects horrific memories, but also visions and memories of community, and these are a strong inducement to stay with the program.

That sense of community created by the war actually made those depressing war years more bearable for many. The adversities at home were endured with more fortitude and sometimes even became laughable. The sadness or grief stemming from the casualties of loved ones on the front lines were mitigated by burgeoning camaraderie at home. Community has immense powers to lessen human travails.

Five years ago, the eminent psychologist David Elkind considered the creeping loss of community from many of our children's schools to be a disaster. The superschool with too many students and too few teachers was providing anonymity instead. The unfortunate result, Elkind said, is that our teenage sons and daughters no longer have a place where they can "construct a sense of who and what they are." After all, a true community is not merely a crowd made smaller. Rather, a community is distinguished by a philosophy that welcomes the particularity of each member and encourages its development. How can a depressed adolescent, who has a pathologically demeaned self-image, reconstruct her identity when in school she has little individuality? A loss of community makes our sons and daughters faceless at school, and faceless against depression.

The junior high or senior high school your teen attends will likely have a profound influence on how he handles the depression. Eric was fortunate. During his first episode, he attended a parochial school in suburban Minneapolis that emphasizes community. My wife and I agreed then, and we agree now, that his depression ran a less ruinous course because of his school. As I conducted the parent interviews for this book, it quickly became clear that most of them spoke of a sense of community at their teen's school as being a substantial modifying factor for the depression.

Besides encouraging individuality, community has several other aspects that are especially relevant for the depressed teen. To explain them, I asked one of the faculty members of Eric's school to discuss in an interview how community may affect a depressed student. Mike Jeremiah is the school's campus minister, the equivalent of a chaplain. He is also a member of the school's Student Support Team, composed of the principal, the guidance staff, the special education teachers, the school's consulting psychologist, and the chemical health counselors.

Q. *How important do you think a sense of community is for a school?*

A. I think community is one of the most important things a school can develop. I think of a community as a "family"—a sense of belonging, a true sense of caring about others, and a concern about how my actions and decisions might affect others. With a sense of community in the school, students support and encourage each other.

Q. *What happens when community is lacking?*

A. Part of community is to notice who is around you. Without it, a depressed student would be more easily lost and fade into the woodwork. In addition, you lose out on self-respect, self-esteem, and you become really susceptible to adverse societal pressures such as provocative dress or drug usage. Life is a search for meaning and something to believe in. In a community we help each other to find that. A lack of community may explain why so many kids get lost so easily. They don't know what the right places are to look in.

Q. *What seems to promote community within a school?*

A. Size is one factor. I really think smaller is better. Another important factor is whether the staff are actually encouraging it. You can tell that by whether teaching for them is more of a job than a vocation. If it's a vocation, they're dedicated.

Q. *What are some of the aspects of school community that you think are especially relevant for a depressed teen?*

A. One is that kids feel comfortable about talking to the adults in the building. They can really connect when they think someone is interested in them. There are many times I learn about a student's problems from other students. I remember a sophomore girl who was very depressed to the point of cutting herself and talking to her friends about wanting to die. I learned about this girl from two of her friends who wanted to talk about it. I don't think this would have happened without the comfort level that community creates. Another important aspect of community is trust among its members. Kids will confide in me. So many times I have been able to call parents about students who I thought were in the early stages of depression that was visible at school but masked at home.

Q. *Any other important aspects?*

A. I think a sense of community fosters mentorship. That's the visible presence of someone who believes in them and offers them something they can believe in. Good example, too. Sometimes I worry we're not offering a lot of that in our society. Some people who profess to be role models are ones I wouldn't pick. The kind of example kids get, whether good or bad, shows them what they have the potential of becoming. Depressed kids need to know their future can be good.

Q. *How can a parent figure out if the school their depressed teen is about to enroll in, or is already attending, is rich in a sense of community?*

A. Obviously, go talk to the principal. Many schools have a Student Support Team like we do, although it might go by a different name. Talk to the head of that team. Also, see if your prospective student can spend the day with a matriculated student. We do that here, and many schools have the same kind of arrangement. One of the very important things to do is to look at what other programs are available besides athletics, routine extracurricular activities, and academic offerings. Are there other activities that will promote personal development? It's not good to become focused on what we are becoming rather than on who we are becoming.

A sense of community in a depressed teen's school promotes that teen's recovery.

Eric is the ultimate proof of my beliefs. Most of the parents I interviewed, too, felt compelled to talk about the importance of community in their teen's school. Belonging to a helpful community that values one's membership erects a formidable defense against the worthlessness and hopelessness that are a depressed teenager's twin demons.

The Supportive School

As I interviewed parents for this book, I was not surprised to discover how strongly they voiced their opinions about the schools their depressed teens were attending. School was the place their teen spent a major portion of the day, and they had decided to become ardent and keen observers of how attending school was affecting the depression. Many of their comments were overwhelmingly positive. The reason was that most of these parents had enlisted the school as a partner with them, and its staff regularly proved to be sympathetic and eager to do all possible to help. I asked these parents where they focused their attention.

Homework. The trend toward more and more homework continues unabated. School boards get pressured by politicians and business leaders to make sure students achieve good grades on standardized tests. Parents begin preparing their children for the SAT and start building their résumés in the sixth or seventh grade.

Homework is a good thing, but not in overload quantities. Yes, homework will improve your teen's performance on standardized tests, but educators who scientifically study homework have determined that too much homework actually turns out to be counterproductive. In fact, some of them have devised a formula to calculate an optimal amount—the "ten-minute rule." For each grade level attained, they say, a child should receive no more than ten minutes of homework each night. According to that rule, a high school senior should have a nightly assignment not to exceed two hours. Not many teachers, parents, or school districts pay heed. Teenagers frequently need to stay up until one or two in the morning to complete lengthy assignments. Or, they may not be completing the assignments at all because their schedules are overbooked with athletic practices, extracurricular activities, or a part-time job.

The result of homework overload is a big dose of stress. "Not doing his homework turns into a tailspin," Dan's mother said. "When he doesn't do the homework, then he doesn't go to class. Then he doesn't take the test. Homework is very stressful for him. Writing a paper sometimes was more than he could bear. He would shut down." Since depression feeds on stress, a parent needs to monitor how much homework her depressed teen is getting. If the load is stressing the teen or the family, both of you should approach teachers at the school to discuss the situation, perhaps diplomatically offering a suggestion for a homework "cap."

Accommodation. "Parents should inform us of the things their child needs," said Bob Tift, the president of the high school Eric attended during his depression. "We want parents to partner with us. Schools want to work together on a solution for the depression just like any special needs situation. Any school is willing to listen, but we would prefer not being dictated to about what to do. When parents get the diagnosis, they should share it with the assistant principal. That's better than talking to the school psychologist, because the psychologist may be attached to the school district, but the principals are right there in the building.

"I know it can be tough to talk because of the stigma, or maybe the parents are reluctant to accept the diagnosis. Maybe there's a factor in the home they don't want to disclose. I would hope they can get over all that. We ask them if they want to talk to their child's teachers. If so, we will arrange a morning meeting for the parent with all of them. If the child has made a suicide attempt, we would like to know about that, too. It might be embarrassing, but the crisis might still be escalating.

"Teachers should make accommodations in homework expectations," Tift said. "We have to keep our priorities straight, don't we?"

Eric had particular difficulty with concentration, a typical symptom of depression. It made every homework assignment a burden. "My reading comprehension was awful," he said, "because I couldn't concentrate. I needed to go over a sentence again and again. You can't learn when you're depressed. I forgot a lot of things during that time."

Katie's mother had nothing but praise for the teachers at Katie's school. "Sometimes she needed to hand something in a day later. Or maybe she needed to take the test later. Don't misunderstand me. I didn't expect any dispensations for anything. One administrator took it upon himself to call all the teachers together with me. We asked Katie if that was okay with her. The one thing that really helped was that all of her teachers knew what was going on, and they were willing to make adjustments."

Extracurricular activities and schedule. It's usually considered a plus if the school encourages participation in a range of extracurricular activities. But too many activities can be stressful. The "overscheduled child" is a worrisome new kind of adolescent. If your teen's schedule is overbooked with all kinds of activities including homework, you might want to log on to an informative Web site, nationalfamilynight.org, created by Dr. Alvin Rosenfeld, a psychiatrist who studies overscheduled children. Read this organization's mission statement. It reminds us that what teens need, especially those who are depressed, is not more activities but more relationships.

There are no set rules for determining how much activity is too much activity. In this context, overscheduling is defined as causing stress. It's all relative. Some teenagers thrive on a busy schedule of extracurricular activities, along with after-school jobs and active social lives. Other teenagers become anxious when they are saddled with too many activities, and the resulting stress can exacerbate the depression. As a parent-partner, you need to periodically examine your teenager's schedule and determine its impact on her emotional health. When necessary, encourage your teen to adjust her schedule to achieve a healthful balance between boredom and overload.

Athletics. If a student's grades are suffering, often the school will take away athletic opportunities. That is counterproductive for a depressed teen. In addition to the biochemical benefits of the exercise, the athletic camaraderie and achievement may be the only bright spot in his day. You may need to step in and be an advocate for your teenager in this area. If you have informed the principal or assistant principal that your teen is dealing with depression, they will usually allow him to continue in athletics despite a poor academic performance.

Tolerance programs for sexual orientation. Last year, the National Mental Health Association surveyed adolescents to determine who were the targets of bullying at school. The results showed that students who were gay or perceived to be gay were the favorite target. Advocacy groups now estimate that 2 million American students are harassed each year because of perceived sexual orientation. It is not uncommon to hear students' language in the dining halls peppered with *dyke* or *fag*.

Programs to train teachers, administrators, and other school personnel about the tolerance of perceived sexual-minority students vary widely by school, school district, and state. If your teen belongs to a sexual minority, be sure to talk to the principal about what programs have been implemented in the school.

Sadly, intolerance may also mean that your teen needs protection, and the principal must answer your questions in this regard. Dan was harassed in the ninth grade by a group of boys who taunted him with shouts of "faggot." "The principal called me about the incident," his mother said. "She was alert to all this. She brought us into her office and said she couldn't promise it would never happen again, but she told me what the school was going to do. They informed the parents of the boys who did it and then suspended them. She informed all of Dan's teachers and the liaison cop on the premises. He met with me and Dan and said he would do whatever it takes to protect him at school. The principal was unbelievably good. I was welcome in her office all the time."

Antibullying programs. That same National Mental Health Association survey identified the other preferred targets for bullying at school. Teens who dressed differently came in second, with obese teens a close third. Disabled teens were next, followed by ethnic minorities, specifically Asians and Latinos.

It's tragic that the majority of teens who get bullied are precisely those who have an inordinate propensity to depression. "He was the tiniest one in his class, and the kids picked on him," Blake's mother said. "He wouldn't tell me that. He was realizing he was different because he didn't look like everyone else. At age thirteen he was becoming isolated. He adopted solitary activities."

Being bullied is so detrimental that the American Medical Association felt compelled to recommend that physicians include questions about it during any pediatric patient visit. It's not just that the victims of bullying can become depressed. They can also become violent. A year after the shootings at Columbine High School, the U.S. Secret Service concluded that most student perpetrators in such shootings had themselves been targets of bullying at school.

A handful of states so far have enacted legislation mandating schools to draw up antibullying policies. To comply with the legal requirement, sometimes a nonprofit organization will offer elementary and middle schools established programs such as "Don't Laugh at Me" or "Names Can Really Hurt Us." Other schools may devise their own plans to fit their specific needs. If your teen is being harassed at school, speak to the principal about what has been put in place to prevent bullying. "My ideal school is [one in which] all kids would be held accountable, including Jared," his mother said.

Caseworker. If you consider your teen's depression to be severe, or if it is complicated by a comorbid condition, ask whether the school could assign a caseworker. "Jared had an advocate who was his caseworker," his mother said. "Anytime I needed to talk, I could call her. It wasn't that way with the principal. He would let Jared down. He told him he would bring him in the office once a week to talk, but he never made good on his promise."

Invisible mentoring. This kind of program goes by different names in different schools. Basically, the teachers identify those students who seem to be lonely, unusually quiet, disconnected, or emotionally distressed. An adult staff member is "assigned" to each one. That person could be a teacher, a member of the administrative staff, or any other adult in the building who is willing to check on that student daily. Invisible mentoring sometimes involves no more than asking, "Did you go to the game last Friday?" or, "Are you making new friends?" The aim is regular adult contact and regular assessment of potential problems. The student generally remains unaware of the "adult assignment" in order to avoid embarrassment in front of peers. If your teen's school doesn't have such a program, ask the principal if there is interest in starting one.

Switching Schools

Should you ever consider switching schools? It's a vexing question because a switch will automatically disrupt your fragile teen's life. Moreover, it can backfire. Mike Jeremiah warned that a switch of schools is sometimes a guaranteed way to make things worse. "A move like that could cause more depression if they have a group of friends that they would be leaving," he said. "I've seen it happen. A switch works only if the kid's open to it. Otherwise, it may cause some rebellion, too."

Of the parents I interviewed, five considered a switch, and two families actually did it. They were well aware of all the caveats that come as slogans: "There are no geographical solutions to intrinsic problems" or "Wherever you go, there you are." Nonetheless, some parents considered their teen's situation at school so unhealthy as to justify considering a switch. Switching schools may make excellent sense when the following situations exist.

Poor fit. "She fit in only to a point," Katie's mother said. "She was afraid to go to school. There was a group of about ten girls [who] were truly bitchy. They were mean. I don't know why, but most of those girls left the school in the tenth grade. When they left, it changed the feel of the whole class. It made space for other people like Katie to do things. I thought a switch [of schools] might make things better because it might allow Katie to make better connections with the kids in her class. Once these girls left, we never did it."

There are many reasons for a poor fit. The school administration may not be generously accommodating to a teen who exhibits the obnoxious behavior of oppositional-defiant disorder. Or the academic offerings may be too rigorous for a teenager with a particularly incapacitating depression. Even if it's a good school, it may be the wrong school for your teenager due to factors you can't change.

Significant family dysfunction. Switching schools may make especially good sense for the anonymous teen at school who has a severely dysfunctional family. An important second part of Dr. Emmy Werner's Kauai study was to focus on which of those two hundred and one "at risk" children turned out to be emotionally healthy despite their family's grim shortcomings. Even with a poor home environment, seventy-two of these children, she said, "grew into competent young adults who loved well, worked well, and played well." One significant protective factor was the school. "They seem to have made school a home away from home," Werner wrote in her scientific reports, "a refuge from a disordered household. When we interviewed them at eighteen, many resilient youths mentioned a favorite teacher who had become a role model, friend, and confidante and was particularly supportive at times when their own family was beset by discord or threatened with dissolution." School was a buffer. Even forty years after their birth, all but two of these seventy-two resilient individuals were doing well in their community. These young people were vulnerable, but invincible, Werner said.

If your teenager is depressed and coping with significant family dysfunction, switching to a better school environment, or to a school that engenders a true sense of belonging, may confer a measure of invincibility.

The current school is too large. School size came up in nearly every interview I had with school administrators and counselors. Many parents concurred. "Roosevelt High was four thousand kids," Alison's stepfather said, "and she felt lost there."

I asked Bob Tift what he would do if his daughter were depressed and attending a large school. "I don't even have to think about that one," he said. "I would send her to a smaller school in a minute. But when that smaller school is a private one, it's an okay decision only if you can afford the tuition."

If the cost of tuition is a concern, know that many private schools charge tuition according to a sliding scale or give outright scholarships based on need. Switching to a different public school is another possibility. "There are wonderful public schools in the [Twin Cities] area, just like in many parts of the country," Tift said. "For economic reasons, school districts have constructed big schools. But many of these big schools are 'made smaller' by establishing 'learning communities' within them. Sometimes it's done by floor, sometimes it's done by class level. It's a difficult thing to pull off, however, but a lot of schools do it."

A parent may object that the learning communities in a depressed child's large school don't seem to function to make the school "smaller." The next step would be to take advantage of the open-enrollment policies many communities have adopted. Depending on the community, you may be able to go to a smaller school in your district or even to a smaller school in a different district. What if that still doesn't seem to provide a satisfactory solution? "I would check into magnet programs," Tift said. "These are sort of learning communities formed around a common theme: for instance, the second language spoken in the home or a particular academic interest."

Single-Gender Schools and Parochial Schools

A single-gender school almost always is smaller, and it might make sense if your teen has huge self-esteem issues. Single-gender schools are harder to find nowadays, but they're worth the search. A single-gender school can be a big help because it is definitely easier to make friends of the same sex. The friendships tend to be lasting, too. Obviously, the student doesn't feel pressured to be popular on campus among the opposite sex.

A single-gender school can be a boost for a girl's self-esteem and academic development, too. No matter how gender-aware we are, in math and science classes, even with women teachers, the boys seem to get called on the most. One of my friends who is an accomplished high school English teacher puts it this way: "Girls get taught early on how to be popular with the boys. One way for sure is not to raise your hand in class." But raising your hand with the right answer promotes self-esteem. A single-gender school doesn't force a girl to choose popularity with the opposite sex over self-esteem.

Parochial schools, whether single- or mixed-gender, should also be considered for the depressed teenager. They offer the advantages of a smaller student body, an emphasis on a sense of community, and more individual attention from the faculty and administrators. In Michelle's case, her father was so certain that a parochial school would be the best environment that he selected a school not affiliated with the family's own religion.

One Size Does Not Fit All

Be aware, however, that small is not the answer for everyone. Your job as the parent-partner is to analyze your teenager's personality and needs to find the school size that fits. Katie's mother is not convinced that size is the crucial issue: "Big is okay if the right people are aware of the child's depression and the child can connect [with other students]. I don't think size is magical."

In fact, Dan and his mother were both delighted when he graduated from a smaller junior high school into a mammoth senior high. Dan had become a target of harassment in junior high because he had made an early gay debut. "There were so many kids in the new school, he welcomed the anonymity," his mother said.

A School Checklist from Parents

Look for these supportive qualities in the junior high or senior high school your teenager attends:
- The school gives your teenager a sense of community.
- Your teenager feels as if she fits or belongs in the school.

- Your teenager's individual qualities are accepted and appreciated by staff and other students.
- Students are encouraged to support each other.
- Students feel comfortable talking to adults in the school.
- Your teenager does not feel overwhelmed or alienated by the school's size.
- The school counseling staff understands teenage depression and has mechanisms in place for recognizing and handling it.
- There is a tolerance program for sexual orientation.
- There is an antibullying program.
- The homework load is manageable.
- There is accommodation for students whose depression is causing academic difficulties.
- Students can participate in athletics even if their grades falter due to depression.

The College Conundrum

When Eric said, "Dad, I want to try going away to college," I was flabbergasted. It was his junior year in high school, and he was just beginning to come out of the depths of his depression. He still couldn't get up in the morning and be on time for classes. My wife and I had to nudge him daily to participate in athletics. He relied on us to plan and involve him in pleasant activities. He relied on us for emotional support. How would he handle any of these things away from home? Perhaps he was just trying to save face by being brave.

I was worried, too. His inner self was rickety. His formula for calculating self-esteem still included big misconceptions. For example, he believed that a person's response to him could only be one of two extremes—complete and unquestioning approval or abject rejection. He was unsure of himself and anxious in new situations. And although his suicide ideation had disappeared, how could I be sure it wouldn't surface again? How would his spirit fare with a sudden deluge of intimidating challenges in a strange place? How could I watch closely when I would be a plane flight away?

To my way of thinking, sending Eric away to college was risky. The downside was obvious and frightening. But, if he could pull it off, the upside was very desirable. Yes, Eric would be forced to cope with unfamiliar circumstances. He would be faced with peculiar or unanticipated problems (his freshman roommate was a nocturnal video-game devotee who seldom attended classes). Eric would have to employ every last ounce of self-discipline he could muster. But if Eric could rise to the challenges, he would learn self-efficacy, and self-efficacy is an antitoxin for the hopelessness of depression. To succeed against some or all of the challenges is like an injection of a miracle drug against depression's worthlessness.

It was worth a try as long as the college was "right" for him. From a distance, I would have to monitor the situation as closely as possible and make sure nothing was going seriously amiss for him. Thank goodness the college he attended had an accommodating calendar of vacations and breaks that allowed Eric to come home every six weeks. My wife or I would visit him on campus in between his trips home. By the time he was ready for his freshman year in college, the depression had resolved. (None of us suspected it would return the following year.)

The kinds of challenges a college presents to a depressed teen and his parents are determined by whether it is a plane ride or a taxi ride away. Which college to choose is a difficult and highly individual decision based on cost, comfort, and the particular emotional deficits your teen has. Some things are not relative, though. For example, persistent suicide ideation or unresolved drug abuse would seem to mandate staying close to home. On the other hand, in the face of serious family dysfunction, or if the teen has a comorbid oppositional-defiant disorder that is fueling family discord, going far away may be the better alternative. The parents and college mental health counselors I interviewed offered these suggestions to help you decide which college might be right for your depressed teen.

Forget the meritocracies. Meritocracies have a difficult time fostering community. Intensely competitive, high-prestige colleges might be entirely inappropriate for a teen who is or was depressed. Everything is earned. Nothing is given. One such university in the Midwest that inordinately emphasizes grades is frequently called "the school that is easier to get into than to get out of." Self-worth is calculated according to grade-point average. That is its culture, and your teen's value is measured by how well he can squeeze himself into that culture. This university also has an alarming suicide rate. In fact, Blake, who had a terrible time fitting into his high school, attended one such meritocracy for two years before he committed suicide.

The meritocracy may not be just an academic one. The intense competition often extends to all kinds of extracurricular activities. There are tryouts for everything. Seldom are there sign-ups, because mere interest or average skills are insufficient to qualify a student for membership. This is the opposite of what you want for an insecure, depressed teen.

You can imagine my delight as I spoke with the water polo coach at the college Eric would be attending. During a chance meeting I mentioned to him that Eric said he might be interested. He asked me if Eric could swim, a remarkable inquiry, since I thought that would be a foregone conclusion. He went on to explain that anyone who wanted to play water polo as a sport at that university could play. It was his mission to create as many squads at as many different skill levels as necessary to accommodate all those students who were interested. No one was excluded, because there were no tryouts. The best of them played in the conference, and they had an admirable record. The worst of them played intramurally, but they still played.

Steer clear of the big schools. Geraldine Rockett is the director of personal counseling and testing at the University of St. Thomas in St. Paul, Minnesota, having earned her Ph.D. in counseling psychology from the University of Pennsylvania twenty-seven years ago. She is also the associate dean of student life and a keen observer of depressed adolescents. "I may be going out on a limb, but I'm going to come down on the side of the small school," she told me. "I wouldn't send a depressed teenager to a school with an enrollment higher than ten to fifteen thousand. In fact, I think the ideal college [for a depressed teen] is one of about one or two thousand students nestled away into the countryside. The small school is where you are more likely to find a nurturing environment."

Look for small class size. All students, especially depressed ones, need to have connections with their professors. The school you are considering should promote small class size and should reward professors for teaching rather than research. Ask the dean or an associate dean if the school routinely solicits letters of recommendation from alumni for their evaluation of a professor's teaching skills as one measure of suitability for that professor's tenure. Professors need to interact with students, because professors are an important safety net for a depressed student.

Avoid the big dormitories. Residence halls should not be twenty-story high-rises. But if there is no choice, they should be divided into smaller units with a resident adviser (R.A.) or a graduate student as an adult on the premises at all times. These people are part of the support network your teen needs, and you should talk to them about the depression if your teen gives you permission. Most college counselors believe the old housemother or housefather idea was great. They say it has gone by the wayside because the "students of the sixties," who are now college administrators, have rejected this idea as too much of an "authoritarian show." No doubt about it, smaller residence halls foster community.

Look into the "first-year experience." Many colleges and universities offer a "first-year experience" program for those students who wish a more familiar introduction to the school and a more friendly living environment for their freshman year. Eric hit the jackpot at his university. The first-year experience placed three hundred freshman students into one residence hall for the entire year. They had their own theater group, band, swimming pool, snack bar, and grocery store. They took many of their required humanities courses together at the dormitory rather than with the student body at large, and they fielded their own intramural athletic teams. They quickly became a cohesive group, and many have kept up their friendships even though they have moved on. "Watch out, though," Dr. Rockett warns. "Some first-year experiences are nothing more than designated groups of students going through orientation together for a day or so."

Check out the counseling center. It should be an identified organization with a director and a full-time counseling staff, not just one person who tries to do everything. The staff should comprise psychologists, social workers, or nurses who are qualified to do mental health counseling and are experienced at it. They should take both the medical and holistic approaches so as to look at a student's strengths in addition to her weaknesses. Check to see how the center's budget is allocated. It makes no sense for the counseling center to employ alcohol- or substance-abuse specialists if equally good resources are available nearby in the community. The money could be better spent on a consulting psychiatrist, for instance, who makes himself readily available for student appointments.

Most of all, the counseling center staff should take a proactive approach. Instead of waiting for students to come to them, they should be pushing out into the residence halls and student unions and presenting programs about mental health issues that students face. In addition, they should take a proactive approach with the faculty. Ask what the counseling center does to educate professors about how to identify a student who is getting into emotional trouble. Also ask if the counseling center conducts such an educational program routinely for new faculty members coming on board.

Counseling centers usually limit the number of visits. Most students are allowed ten to fifteen per year. Ask what happens if your teen needs more visits than the center allows.

Log on to the counseling center's Web site. Most counseling centers have them. "Ours has all the screening tools, such as inventories which assess depression, anxiety, eating disorders, alcohol abuse, or suicide ideation," Dr. Rockett said. "That's the beauty of the Internet. More students and parents check us out than ever before."

An excellent resource for college students and concerned parents is provided by the Jed Foundation, an organization committed to reducing the young-adult suicide rate and improving mental health support for college students. Their Web site, www.jedfoundation.org, offers links to "Ulifeline" Web sites that provide mental health information, education, and student self-screening.

It's Not All Academics

Basically, what Dr. Rockett and the other counselors I interviewed were saying is that the school ought to be a community. It ought to discern, value, and make a special place for its members. And its members ought to watch out for each other.

Dr. Rockett finished up the interview with these comments: "If your student is a star tennis player, and the tennis team at the college you are looking at is no good, why would you send your child there? If you had a child in a wheelchair, why would you send her to a college that is not wheelchair-accessible, no matter how good it is academically?"

Think about it. Perhaps the school's academic standing ought not to be the ultimate criterion. Community deserves that first-place consideration.

Part 3

Stay the Watch

Recovery, Recurrences, and Building Resilience

13

Ups and Downs

As a surgeon, in my particular specialty of medicine, I cared for patients who had cancers of the throat or jaw. With the tools of modern surgery and radiation therapy, many of them were cured, but sometimes they would come out of it all with serious deficits of speech or swallowing. Even before they had been discharged from the hospital, even before their incisions had completely healed, therapists were visiting their rooms and intensively teaching them how to compensate for the loss of a voice box or for the terrible difficulty of choking as swallowed food usually "got down the wrong pipe." It's called rehabilitation. It's meant to undo as much of the damage or to offset as many of the deficits as possible from the despoilment of that terrible disease. Doctors have matured enough in their thinking about cancer of the head and neck to consider cosmesis an indispensable part of rehabilitation, too. A resulting facial deformity should not go unattended and cause a patient to be embarrassed by his appearance and stay away from friends, clubs, and shopping malls. Reconstructive-plastic surgeons are recruited into the team right away. Deformities are camouflaged or undone.

Besides cancer, we rehabilitate patients with many other kinds of diseases, and for all kinds of reasons. Some of these diseases are terrible, such as multiple sclerosis or stroke, and we feel the humane need to go all out. Some of them are much less severe but disabling, such as carpal tunnel syndrome, and rehabilitation gets the patient back to work. Some of them are athletic conditions, and we don't want to miss out watching our favorite players on Monday nights or Sunday afternoons. Some are even uniformly fatal, such as Alzheimer's disease. Despite impending death, though, we want to provide these unfortunate people as many days of "intactness" as possible.

We rehabilitate patients with these diseases because they leave an aftermath. I've never seen the word *aftermath* used in a good context. There's no such thing as an aftermath of a wedding or a celebration, unless, of course, bottles were heaved or a guest was punched. There is, however, an aftermath of a tornado, a war, a violent hurricane, or an awful disease. Like cancer or a stroke, depression leaves behind its own brutal aftermath. People who have been depressed say that the consequences of depression will determine the rest of their life. This is indeed the case.

So, where are the rehabilitation programs and specialists to address the after-effects of depression? They are few and far between.

One of the handful of such programs is Boston University's Center for Psychiatric Rehabilitation. In existence for over twenty years, the center offers individual and group services for adolescents and adults who have experienced psychiatric illness. "It's a safe place where people can start thinking about what they want to do and build confidence," says Kerri Hamilton, coordinator of services.

"Self-confidence is such a big piece. There aren't many [such rehabilitation centers], although there are so many parallels to a physical disability."

That's where you, the parent-partner, come in.

The task defaults to the parents to be the primary rehabilitation therapists for their depressed teen after recovery. Because of having gone through the maelstrom herself, surely your teen will be an inventor and initiator of part of the rehabilitation effort. But she still risks getting buffeted in depression's wake, because an adolescent is an inexperienced thinker and planner. You make up for these deficiencies of her youth. You have love, and moreover, you have wisdom. You will have to observe and counsel her.

On what should you train your sights? I've compiled a list of aftermath factors that seem to affect three important aspects of life: interior life, personal life, and economic life. This information comes from what depressed people themselves have experienced, and from what parents had to say about their children once the depression had passed.

Interior Life

Constant uncertainty and fear. Depressed people say that when the gray cloud of melancholy blows in, no matter how small or wispy, the immediate fear is that it does not represent mere sadness but heralds the thunderhead of depression. They panic when they sense a downturn in mood, because the downturn may represent the start of another inexorable slide into the void. They need always to remind themselves, and to have others such as a parent remind them when their conviction falters, of a crucial distinction. Sadness can easily be identified because it leaves hope intact. Sadness means that your really funny friend will seem funny again tomorrow. It means that a really juicy hamburger will be delectable one day soon. In depression, however, everything seems permanently bland and empty, with no believable prospects that anything will change for the better. Depression dashes hope and in its place weaves despair.

People who used to be depressed are always scanning for any blip of emptiness. At strange hours, Eric would call me from college—sometimes frankly worried, sometimes trying in vain to disguise a terror—about his mood. "I've been down for two days," he would say. "What does this mean? Is it normal? Should I start back on medicines?" Thank goodness he often had enough composure to reassure himself by falling back on the precise medical definition of depression. Sometimes, though, I had to coach him hard. Often the next day he would call back and say that the mood had passed. "I was just bummed out by a chemistry exam, and I'm okay now." I could hear the relief, almost joy, in his voice, and his resolve to press on, because another week or month had passed without the return of the scourge. I knew, however, another such phone call was not long off, and I would have to be available and ready for a long conversation.

Some people can't be analytical like Eric, the chemistry major, because that's not the way they prefer to process information. Instead, in defense against the terrifying feeling, they numb themselves and become detached. If I don't allow myself to feel anything, they reason, it might be impossible for me to feel depressed. The danger here is that the persistent detachment may turn into an emotional handicap called alexithymia. People with this condition have lost the ability to recognize specific emotions in themselves and in others. These unfortunate people have little empathy, little interest in others, and little interest in sexual activity.

A person who has experienced an episode of depression lives in fear he will not be able to soothe himself when his world starts quaking. This is the reason self-control and self-efficacy are such crucial talents for a depressed person to cultivate. They get him out of a jam. That is why parents must encourage a rigorous approach to self-control and continually remind their teens of their successes in extricating themselves from all kinds of emotional difficulties.

Secrecy. To whom, if ever to any person, should a teen admit she had been depressed? To a new boyfriend, or to the boyfriend's parents, to prove that no matter what either of them heard, everything is all right now? How about to a new college roommate, to make excuses ahead of time in case anything "peculiar" happens during the school year? The sad truth is that many listeners won't "buy into this whole depression business." As a result, most depressed people become convinced it is best to conceal it all. Living with a secret is taxing. But many teens would rather live with the secret than with the stigma.

Many teens have imperfect physical health. Luke, the son of our friends from Seattle, has perforated eardrums. His ears discharge, and his hearing is poor. His brother, Jeff, has a recurring dislocated shoulder, brought on by too many crushing blocks while playing on his high school football team's offensive line. Patrick, the son of neighbors down the street, has juvenile-onset diabetes and gives himself daily insulin injections. These young people tell me about their problems, and their parents tell me, too. They don't have much of a secret, because there isn't much of a stigma.

Then, too, I don't think many adolescents have perfect emotional health. The adage is true: the only normal people are the ones you don't know so well. Emotional illness is the family secret everyone has. As I interviewed parents for this book, they usually considered it safe to talk. They would let the secret out not only about their depressed teenagers, but also about their other children, who had different emotional problems. So, why should problems of emotional health condemn a teen to some kind of secret and disparaged subgroup, when seldom does that happen with problems of physical health? The truth is that people have preconceived notions about sanity and madness. There's supposed to be a continuum, they say, and they place depression somewhere on this scale between these two extremes. The degree of depression, therefore, must correspond to the degree of madness. I would offer that it doesn't belong on this scale at all, just as it is inappropriate to place chicken pox or acne somewhere on the continuum between malignant disease and benign disease. More pox or more pimples doesn't imply a greater tendency to malignancy. But here is the fundamental question: In conscience, how can we ever justify stigmatizing any form of human suffering, physical or emotional, and especially when the suffering is so great? The only help parent-partners can give their teens in this regard is to beat down the stigma. They must also not subscribe to the stigma themselves.

Guilt. Many teens want to do penance and make restitution for the aloofness, anger, or misbehavior that occurred during the throes of the depression. Eric hated everything about high school, and he graduated thinking it was all his fault. He saddled himself with guilt even though he couldn't have controlled much about the situation. Only now can he look back wistfully and realize high school could have been better—if only circumstances beyond his control had been better. It is a parent's responsibility to help a formerly depressed teen look back with objectivity. From our past, we all have accumulated enough legitimate baggage to tote around without needing to add to that burden any unjustified parcels.

A fractured relationship with the Creator. In her book about depression, *On the Edge of Darkness,* author Kathy Cronkite said it this way: "Depression is a distorted and pessimistic view of the world, from which our relationships to Eternity are not exempt." Like cancer, the suffering is so great and so purposeless that it seems as if whatever God there is must certainly have abandoned the depressed person. Moreover, the God may be viewed as malevolent, conjuring the blasphemous prayer "Forgive me for my little jokes on thee, and I will forgive thy great big one on me." Some parents of depressed teens who have committed suicide feel their child must have concluded, in spite of a devout faith, that God had abandoned or was punishing him or her before embarking on that final act. I must be so worthless, these teens must have said to themselves, that even the deity has cursed me. Thus, rescue will be impossible. There is no reason to carry on. Once the depression lifts, however, remorse sets in for shaking a fist to the sky.

Personal Life

Fractured relationships with teachers, friends, and siblings. Once the depression lifts, a teen often looks back and sees innumerable lost and damaged relationships. She may have alienated her teachers with missed assignments, flimsy excuses, unexcused absences, and belligerence in the classroom. Her friends may have been offended by what they thought was her aloofness when she was actually scared, her terseness when she was actually anxious, her peculiar behavior when she just couldn't think of anything to say, or her inability to accept a hug because she felt unlovable. Now, in the aftermath, her friends may not want to hear from her because she offended them so often when she was a mess. People may be uncomfortable around her if they know she attempted suicide. At home, her brothers and sisters may have been relegated to second-class shadow siblings because she got most of her parents' attention.

A satisfactory repair of many of these damaged relationships may be impossible. Unflattering impressions of the depressed teen may be fixed in people's minds, and in some cases no amount of extra care now will totally compensate for the past interpersonal difficulties. Worse yet, explaining that the bad behavior was all due to depression may undo many of the misperceptions, but at the expense of stigmatization. Parents would likely be wise to counsel their teens that, in many cases, it is better not to attempt any repairs at all and concentrate rather on moving forward. In fact, scientific studies indicate that that may indeed be the most sensible plan. Once the depression resolves, adolescents routinely enjoy just as wide a circle of friends, and just as much contact with them, as people who were not depressed as teens. Yet, there is always profound sadness in leaving the bygones as displeasing bygones. The opportunities for human contact that were missed or bungled will never be had to do over. It is a hard lesson even for most adults to accept.

Enduring personality changes. Anyone who says that a person's predepression personality rebounds unscathed has never been depressed. Much of it does, but it returns crumpled, with permanent and undesirable wrinkles. Most young people are naturally upbeat, but depression stomps hard on their optimism. They often come out of the depression cynical, or frequently suspicious that things won't work out well for them. They consider Thoreau irrelevant or foolish because he exhorts his reader "to go confidently down the path of your dreams, and live the life you've imagined." They know they have been struck down by circumstances not of their own making, and they were unable to get up under their own power. They imagine a future of again trying to rise from their knees.

Their charming if naive quality of omnipotence gets more than tempered. They were not masters over the depression, and their sense of self-efficacy was smashed. As a consequence, they may develop dependent personality traits. Eric still inordinately looks to me to help him select college courses, careers, even a car. It's more than just politely asking the advice of an elder. It's a stunning lack of confidence in his own very real powers. Dependency stifles the development of self-efficacy—and that can become a vicious circle.

If you thought that your daughter was a natural-born leader, depression will likely stifle her leadership abilities. How can she believe that others will adhere to her opinions and follow them when she is desperately trying to recapture the capacity to believe in herself? Winston Churchill and Abraham Lincoln were strongly effective leaders despite their spasms of depression. I have no doubt, though, that they were the rare and exceptional survivors of the disease, and I am troubled when I wonder how great is the number of capable young leaders we have lost to teenage depression.

Hedonism. Some formerly depressed people turn hedonistic. They use the constant pursuit of pleasurable activities as a counteroffensive against an invasion of sadness or despair. In truth, this approach is nothing more than an opiate. It prevents the formerly depressed person from confronting any disconcerting emotional issue head-on. If nothing pleasurable is available to latch onto, perhaps something can be manufactured in which to rejoice. Conjuring delight from the mundane, or brilliance from the gloom, becomes a protective habit, albeit hocus-pocus. Maybe if I always laugh, maybe if I always strain to see the lively side, the depression can't sneak back in.

Marriage difficulties. Adolescent depression seems to exert no effect whatsoever on ultimate marriage rates. There is no increased probability of remaining single as a young adult. But these statistics don't necessarily signify eventual marital success.

More than one scientific study has documented that young women who were depressed as adolescent girls marry at an earlier age than women who had never been depressed. This is so for various reasons. For one thing, the dependency that a past depression breeds often increases the need to have a partner in a significant relationship. Also, some depressed girls have ongoing conflicts with their parents, as did Michelle, which hasten the leaving of the family of origin. Lastly, depression can destroy a person's ability to achieve intimacy, and early marriage often represents an ongoing cry for intimacy. This may well be the reason also that these young women have more children. Children represent an attempt by a formerly depressed woman to increase her sense of connectedness to others. Children provide instant intimacy and a social network.

Although early marriage may actually turn out to be a solution to some of the aftermath of depression, for young women it comes with significant costs. Early marriage often portends increased marital instability, greater child-care burdens, reduced economic resources, and curtailed educational attainment.

Sadly, both young men and young women who had been depressed as adolescents later report decreased marital satisfaction. They get involved in more marital disagreements, especially the young men, and especially those of both genders who had experienced comorbid anxiety disorders. But a past depression also usually intrudes into a marriage in more insidious ways. For many, an adolescent depression will forever impair the achievement of emotional closeness. Indeed, studies document less closeness with a marriage partner or a marriagelike partner, perhaps owing to unresolved negative or unfriendly social behavior that the depression fostered. Some of the difficulties are a "carryover phenomenon." In other words, these young people reproduce within their marriages the same types of interpersonal difficulties they frequently experienced with their parents. Lastly, some psychologists think that depressed people tend to marry other depressed people—and then the marriage gets a double dose of the aftermath.

This rather harsh account of marital outcomes may prove in a decade or so to be inaccurate, as this picture is based on the best scientific studies available today. Today's long-term follow-up study of young people who had been depressed ten or more years ago when they were adolescents usually means they were treated before the availability of the newer antidepressants, such as the SSRIs. Rather, they had been treated in the eighties with the earlier-generation drugs that we now know were quite ineffective. Moreover, at that time, they likely were not treated as aggressively, because adolescent depression was just beginning to be recognized as a genuine disease. Many doctors were still doubters, hesitant to go full tilt against it. Thus, we haven't yet calculated the marital outcomes for teens who have gotten modern, intensive, and comprehensive treatment. Even today, however, some psychologists and psychiatrists still predict that we will eventually see an increased divorce rate among those who were depressed as adolescents. Perhaps that may prove true only for those who were treated inadequately.

As your teen's primary rehabilitation partner, you should counsel her on how to choose a "significant other" for marriage or a marriagelike arrangement. Don't feel guilty. You're not arranging a marriage. You're only trying to help her avoid the shoals. Continue to ask her physician about new studies of marital outcome, or download them after a search on PubMed. One warning. Despite the current scientific omens, don't ever dissuade your previously depressed teen from getting married to the right person. Instead, actively encourage it. A good marriage with a carefully chosen partner may not only lead to a lifetime of loving companionship but also be a powerful prescription for a previously depressed teen. In fact, a study of over two thousand twin pairs conclusively showed that marriage, or a marriagelike relationship, significantly decreased the impact of the inherited genetic predisposition to depression. A good marriage can overcome even the power of genes, and it may protect against recurrences. Strong medicine indeed.

Physical health. People who have been depressed seem to get more angina and more heart attacks. No pathological mechanism has yet been discovered to explain this curious statistic. Perhaps depression simply encourages poor self-care, such as overeating, smoking, or decreased adherence to medications, or perhaps, on a more fundamental level, it actually promotes or worsens narrowing of the heart's coronary arteries.

It might be easier to explain why depressed people get more

infections, since depression has been documented to reduce the capacities of the immune system. The same perturbation of the body's immune functions may be responsible for the observed increase in deaths from breast cancer and malignant melanoma among people who have been depressed. Some immunologic processes are important in the defense against the development or progression of certain kinds of cancer. In fact, people who are depressed or subjected to severe stress—a prelude to depression—show immune deficiencies. Studies of depressed hospitalized patients, lonely persons, bereaved or caregiving spouses, and even college students taking final exams reveal important deficits of anticancer surveillance mechanisms. Further research must clarify whether the observed deficits are of sufficient type and magnitude to explain accelerated tumor growth. The jury is still out.

Anxiety disorder. Even teens who did not have a comorbid anxiety disorder with their depression face an outsize risk for developing this second emotional illness. The statistics seem to show that a previously depressed teen has twice the chance of eventually developing an anxiety disorder as a nondepressed teen. Go back to chapter 5 and review the symptoms of anxiety disorders so that you can take this watch.

Economic Life

Employment. Dr. Steve Miles has an office several doors down from mine at the University of Minnesota's Center for Bioethics. An intelligent and empathetic physician, Dr. Miles was the subject of a lengthy *New York Times* article in July 2003 that told how he became acutely depressed and contemplated suicide a few years ago. He quickly sought treatment, got the illness to remit, and never missed a day's work through it all. The trouble with his job began afterward when he applied to the Minnesota Board of Medical Practice to renew his medical license. The application form asked whether he had been "treated for any nervous or mental condition." He replied truthfully, and his application was promptly rejected. Dr. Miles was incensed because he felt just as capable of practicing medicine as he did before the illness struck, an opinion unanimously shared by his colleagues. And so, he took upon himself the huge task of having the board change its application to ask instead whether the person was "*impaired* because of any nervous or mental condition."

The stigma attached to depression—its persistence and unfairness—is the point of his story. Until only recently, the official position of the board was that the mere diagnosis of depression was sufficient to disqualify a person from practicing medicine. But Dr. Miles is absolutely right. The real arbiter ought to be impairment. Diabetes, for example, shouldn't disqualify one for work, but diabetes resulting in impaired vision rightly may, depending on the nature of the job. Many employers have not yet come around to this way of thinking, and many will not until they are coerced. That's why many previously depressed people are forced to hide their diagnosis. A bigger sadness occurs if their depression strikes again. To avoid discovery, these people often avoid treatment. Thus, the stigma that denies these people employment may also work to make the disease worse.

What does a history of depression portend once these teens start on a career and get a job? Although they may have to work around the stigma problem, thankfully the disease itself does not confer a risk at all of becoming "underemployed." Teens with a history of depression succeed in getting hired into just as rewarding and prestigious occupations as those who have never been depressed, and they earn just as good an income. The only exception occurs when the depression had been especially severe, and when the teen winds up with relatively poor educational attainment. These individuals experience both underemployment and unemployment.

Insurance. After being treated for an emotional illness, a teen may eventually have to fight to obtain various kinds of insurance. The hardest kind to obtain is long-term disability insurance. Many carriers will automatically disqualify an applicant with any kind of psychiatric history. Health insurance usually is obtainable if your teen is a part of a group plan. Federal law bars discrimination against any individual in a group plan, and insurers don't worry about the particular risks of individual members when the group is large. But if your teen becomes self-employed, for example, and thus is not part of a group, the situation can be difficult. The more serious the depression, and especially with bipolar disorder, the greater is the likelihood an individual applicant will face disqualification. Life insurance is the easiest kind to obtain, but a previously depressed person may not get the lowest "preferred" premium rates offered to healthy nonsmokers. It pays to shop around for insurance. Each insurance company formulates its own underwriting guidelines based on how much money people with a history of depression have cost the company in the past year. If a particular insurer has had a good experience with previously depressed people, your teen may be able to obtain insurance at favorable rates.

Types of Recurrences

There are two ways of calculating the health burden of a disease for an individual. One is to calculate the number of years of life lost owing to a premature death. The second way makes more sense because it adds to this number also the number of years the person lived with any disability due to the disease. Using this kind of calculation, the World Health Organization, in collaboration with the World Bank, estimated what the global burden of depression would be in the years to come. The result is shocking. Depression will rank second—not accidents, stroke, lung diseases, cancer, or even the injuries from violence and war. Only heart disease will inflict a greater health burden than depression on the peoples of the world.

Depression ranks ominously because it is now correctly being looked upon as a recurrent disorder. The recurrences, which may turn out to be frequent, account for the great number of years a person must live with disabilities. With each episode come functional disruptions just as devastating as those of tuberculosis or diabetes, and the disruptions widely affect a person's employment, student work, household duties, recreation, satisfaction, and relationships with family and friends.

None of the scientists who have studied adolescent depression have yet conclusively identified the factors that increase a teen's chances for a recurrent, second episode. Still, the sum of their studies provides a useful, though provisional, checklist for parents. Their list includes suicide ideation or suicide attempt, comorbid dysthymia, being female, low socioeconomic status, or a severe first episode. Any of these factors may mean your teen is headed for another crash.

These scientists calculations for a second episode are only approximations, but the range of their predictions is alarming. Some investigators say the odds are no less than fifty-fifty. Others go to an extreme, saying the chances are as high as 90 percent. Many of these studies show that about 50 percent of previously depressed teens will suffer a second episode within three years, and that about 70 percent will do so within five years.

If the depression recurs, it usually comes back in one of two forms.

Major depressive disorder. This is likely what happened to your teen the first time. Go back to chapter 4 and review the diagnostic criteria to see if they fit again. An additional worry is that what you are observing may turn into what some psychiatrists call *rapid cycling* or *cycle acceleration*. These terms mean that each recurrent episode will become more severe, more frequent, and more treatment-resistant than the previous episode.

This phenomenon is a worry, but with the involvement of a parent-partner, it is not an inevitability. The first thing you must do is to hunker down and consider that your teen's depression will likely be a lifetime disorder. The cited high recurrence rates should convince you of this. If you maintain this posture, you will maintain your vigilance. At the slightest suspicion of recurrence, ask your teen about his mood, his anxiety, and his worries. Also, check with your teen's doctor to see if resumption of the antidepressants or psychotherapy seems warranted. If you are going to make a mistake, make it in the direction of overtreatment. With antidepressants being so safe, the risks of overtreatment are fairly slim, but undertreatment may be catastrophic.

Eric was getting unjustifiably cranky during his first summer home from college. I didn't wait for any other symptoms. He and I chatted heart-to-heart. He admitted the depression might be returning, and he resumed taking antidepressants for over a year, and with gratifying results. Prompt and decisive action on your part can save the day. Early and aggressive treatment of the second episode can decrease the chances of a third.

Despite the foreboding statistics, your teen has a real chance to escape the ravages of recurrences and cycle acceleration. With a second or third episode, even if it gets treated to full resolution, you should feel bound to ask your teen's doctor about lifelong medication for him.

Recurrent brief depression. This European name hasn't quite caught on in the United States, although the concept was accepted by American psychiatrists years ago. This kind of recurrent depression started off being called *intermittent depressive disorder,* then *very brief depressions,* and then *intermittent three-day depressions,* until the term *recurrent brief depression* (RBD) was adopted.

RBD is not a lesser disease for being "brief." It is the full-blown clinical picture of depression. The symptoms are precisely the same as with a major depressive episode. The differences lie in the duration of the symptoms and the frequency of their recurrence. Typically, RBD episodes last for two or three days and occur about once per month for at least a year. It's remarkably easy to set off episodes. They may be triggered by mild stressors or may even occur spontaneously. (In females, the episodes do not occur only in relation to the menstrual cycle, as is the case with PMS.) Attesting to the severity of RBD is that the total number of depressed days a person with this disease will experience in a lifetime is about the same as that of someone with a recurrent major depression. Moreover, the rate of suicide attempts is higher. This form of depression is insidious. It often goes unrecognized because the short duration of the symptoms often prevents recognition by a physician. It is adequately treated with medications less than 20 percent of the time, even though it may be one of the most common types of recurrent depression. The biggest danger is that the sufferer often trivializes it as "nothing more than a monthly case of the blues that will pass." As a parent-partner, you must be especially vigilant for this kind of recurrence. The long-term suffering and dangers are no less than with major depression.

Crashing in College

As I've mentioned, statistics indicate that 70 percent of the recurrences happen within five years of the first episode, which means that one may occur while your son or daughter is still attending school.

Recurrent depression doesn't have its own calendar, however. It follows the calendar of the stresses your teen encounters. If the first episode occurred in middle or junior high school, the transition to a strange and often intimidating high school is no picnic for a teen's psyche. If your teen became depressed before high school, the statistics emphasize how important the choice of an appropriate high school will be. Go back to chapter 12 and review the criteria for the optimal school.

If your teen's first episode occurred in senior high school, then often the recurrence will come in college, as it did for Eric. The demands of attending college have always made it a stressful place, but the last decade has added new and dangerous stressors. Many college students are trying to amass credentials that attest to their energy and intelligence by electing double majors. In 2002, for example, 23 percent of Georgetown University graduates and 42 percent of Washington University liberal arts graduates had pursued double majors, all in an attempt to be more competitive in the job market or for a presumed better chance at admission to graduate or professional schools. That's not the worst of it. Some saddle themselves with triple and quadruple majors. Parents seem to be encouraging the trend, but many professors think it gives the student no substantial competitive edge worth the effort. The burgeoning economic burden of attending college has become an important new stressor as tuition soars and financial aid shrinks. If a student must work his way through college, the routine can be punishing. A recent survey showed that fully three-quarters of full-time undergraduate students now work, putting in an average of twenty-five hours each week. Even the once appealing "junior year abroad" is turning out to be less of an adventure and more of a stressor. Documented now is that increasing numbers of students are spending the year overseas cultivating stress by experimenting with drugs or getting pregnant. It's not unusual for some of them to return home depressed.

Dr. Geraldine Rockett, who offered such good advice on choosing a college, also had insights into dealing with depression on campus.

Q. *Is depression common in college students?*

A. Very much so. It's always in the top two or three conditions which college counseling centers see students for.

Q. *What precipitates depression in college students?*

A. A bunch of things. They're in a lot of transitions. Their parents and friends will tell them these are the best years of their lives, but they've forgotten how bad it really was—living away from home, living with a stranger, taking difficult courses, and you can't get up in the middle of the night for a meal. Adolescents have higher highs and lower lows, and this makes things more devastating. Most of them don't have extended families nearby. A lot of kids work to pay the bills. Some of our students go to class, do an internship, and have a job—all at the same time. It could be a real source of stress that precipitates a depression, but it depends on the student.

Q. *How about relationships?*

A. When people come in for counseling, often it's because a boyfriend or girlfriend dumped them. Depression can follow. For the boys, often it's been a long-standing relationship, and they don't have much else going on besides school. The girl provided all the emotional support and connections. Their friends get tired of hearing about their problems, so they come to the counseling center.

Q. *Which years have the most depression?*

A. Freshman year because of the transitions—there's always something new. Sophomore year is bad, too, because the novelty is over, and [students] realize that there is a lot of hard work to be done.

Q. *May a depressed college student take a medical leave without jeopardizing his grade point average?*

A. It depends on how formal the college or university is. You may get an I [incomplete] or a W [withdrew] for your courses, and that shouldn't hurt your grade point average. But at some schools, you could get an F if it's during the last two weeks of the semester and you haven't gotten a letter from a psychologist at the counseling center. That will definitely affect your grade point. Some schools take a very human view. They believe that the student and the family are in the best position to make the decision about what kinds of grades ought to appear on the transcript. On the other hand, some schools make it hard to get back in after leaving for mental health issues. They make you jump through a lot of hoops. It's best for parents to look into these things ahead of time.

Q. *Should a student who was depressed in high school check in with a personal counselor like you as soon as freshman classes begin?*

A. Yes, especially if they don't have a counselor at home. I would immediately ask them if they wanted to start a counseling relationship here. The usual scenario is that the parent approaches me first. I then ask the parent to talk to the student to encourage him or her to scope us out on our [counseling] Web site.

Q. *How do the professors at your university accommodate to a depressed student?*

A. Because of confidentiality, we can't notify professors that a student is depressed and ask them to make adjustments. If the student establishes a counseling relationship, a psychologist will ask him to sign a release for the dean's office and encourage the student to talk to his professors.

They will have to do that anyway if the depression gets in the way of their studies. The beauty of a smaller school like ours is that there are many other ways of working with a student. The [dormitory resident adviser] usually knows about the depression anyway, and so does the dean of student life. In a small school, it gets known through the grapevine, and that's how the safety net gets thrown up.

Q. *What about the issue of confidentiality as it affects parents?*

A. My goal is to get a support network in place for the student, not to get the parents informed. During orientation, we encourage parents to call the counseling center. We talk to them about how confidentiality issues restrict what kinds of information we can give out to them.

Q. *What is your philosophy about the school assuming some of the protective duties of the parents while their child is on campus? The legal terminology is* in loco parentis.

A. I take the middle ground. It makes no sense to go back to the days of housemothers and signing in and out. However, the pendulum has swung too far the other way. Students unfortunately have minimal contact with adults. Often it's only with their professors, and then only in class. After classes, sometimes there are no adults around. We shouldn't be holding their hands, but throwing them into the abyss is not right either. They're still kids in many ways.

Q. *When would you advise a student to switch to a college closer to home?*

A. If they're not making friends, getting connected, or doing well academically. The critical factor, however, is whether they have a good support network here at school. Home might not turn out to be what they expect. None of their friends might be there because they're all scattered away at different colleges.

Q. *How should parents communicate with a depressed child who is away at college?*

A. I ask them to set up a plan before they [drop their child off at school] and return home. I ask the kid what he wants. Some will want an e-mail three or four times a day, and they will want them answered right away, too. Others will want a phone call every night. Visits during parents' weekends are a must.

The Job Crunch

Some high school graduates will go straight to the job market, and that move may prove sufficient to trigger a recurrence. There is now more stress here, too. School psychologists have estimated that career-related anxieties have increased at least 20 percent in the last few years. The reason has been the recent economic downdraft. We've gone from reading about teenage millionaires who got started in their garage to reading about bankrupt parents who have lost their savings in a plummeting stock market. In your job-seeking teen's mind, economic optimism may have been replaced by economic angst. Don't believe that your child is immune to such "adult" concerns. The future has always been very much on the minds of high school students. Just ask your son or daughter. You might be surprised to hear how intense are their worries about ever finding a good job.

Finding the right job after getting a college degree is equally, if not more, stressful. Dr. Rockett notes, "The 'umbilical cord' gets cut when they leave college. A lot of kids have been grooming themselves for a particular job over four years. Then, they can't get a job that's even close. It's stressful because it's frustrating."

Postpartum Depression

Giving birth may be another triggering event for a recurrence. The birth of a child is an enormous joy mixed with enormous stress, and the odds of a young woman developing postpartum depression are about one in eight. Hormone deficiencies are important root causes for this mysterious emotional illness. Psychosocial factors share much of the responsibility. If the new mother has had an episode of adolescent depression, the odds for postpartum depression seem to increase dramatically to about one in three. The symptoms occur within six months of delivery. Not only does the mother suffer, but the consequences for the infant can be equally severe and include alienation, indifference, resentment, and hostility. If this results in failure to bond with the child, then significant problems persist long after resolution of the depression.

What can you as a parent-partner do to prevent postpartum depression? Not much, I'm afraid, at least according to the most recent scientific literature. All you can do is watch your daughter closely, especially if she has some of the other risk factors. These include marital problems, depression during pregnancy, complications during delivery, and either you or your spouse having been depressed yourselves. Further research is needed to devise a screening tool to reliably identify the women at the highest risk and to figure out ways of preventing their likely postpartum depression. But your vigilance, and encouraging your daughter to seek treatment promptly, will stave off depression's harm from a child and a grandchild.

14

Partnering: The Path to Refuge and Resilience

Everything about the human body ought to have a purpose. When the purpose of an organ, an enzyme, or a brain function continues to elude scientists, they get extremely nervous.

One reason for their worry is that the purposeless component may actually be some kind of mischievous hanger-on, such as the appendix. A vestigial structure fashioned in eons gone by, it was somehow useful to our prehistoric ancestors. Today, however, it seems to do nothing positive for our fragile existence, and evolution hasn't yet gotten around to discarding it. To our detriment, it can behave badly despite our hospitality, much like an uninvited relative who complains about the dinner and the guest room. In a cantankerous mood, it can inflict bad belly pain and a high fever, necessitating an emergency appendectomy, usually at an inconvenient hour.

But the far bigger cause for scientists' worry is that they still aren't being clever enough to discover the intentions of that seemingly purposeless thing. The year I took an immunology course as an undergraduate student, scientists were literally staying up nights worrying about the lymphocyte, a microscopic blood cell described in my assigned textbook as "functionless." Because the only known behavior of this enigmatic cell was occasionally to mutate into lymphocytic leukemia or a malignant lymphoma, one view was that the lymphocyte was nothing more than a mischievous ne'er-do-well. There was a problem with that line of thought. I only had one appendix, but I had billions of these unimposing and homely cells flowing with my blood, and percolating throughout all of my organs. I was awash in lymphocytes. Why the huge numbers? On top of that, as the older lymphocytes died off, my body saw fit to immediately produce young and vigorous replacements. Why wouldn't my body let the numbers dwindle?

Ten years after my immunology course, scientific journals were becoming crammed with reports of yet another newly discovered function for these benevolent cells. The excitement in the medical community was so great that the National Institutes of Health was awarding research fellowships to encourage all sorts of young scientists to take up their study. I received one of these fellowships and spent the next four years at the Sloan-Kettering Institute investigating one of the many subfunctions of these invaluable cells in the body's defense against cancer. It was turning out that lymphocytes also staunchly protected us against all kinds of bacterial, viral, and fungal infections. They were a blood-borne flying squadron of well-trained and ferocious defenders. So significant was the discovery of the many purposes of lymphocytes that my mentor at Sloan-Kettering, Dr. Robert A. Good, received this country's Lasker Award, sometimes a prelude to the Nobel Prize. In elucidating the crucial functions of these "functionless cells," he figured out how he could perform the first bone-marrow transplant, and the recipient is alive today. We all cheered him when his picture appeared on the cover of *Time* magazine on March 19, 1973. I didn't have a hint a decade earlier, when I was reading my immunology textbook, that any of this was going to happen.

All the workings of the brain should have a purpose, too. The brain permits us to feel pain, and it is easy to figure out why. If our shins didn't sting after bumping them on the sideboards when we remade the bed linens, bumping them repeatedly would lead to skin ulcers on the fronts of our legs right down to the bone. We quickly learn not to bump. Painful blisters tell us to wear better shoes the next time we go running, and a burned hand tells us to use an oven mitt when retrieving the pizza. Fear is also easy to figure out. A decidedly unpleasant emotion, fear will cause us to take a foot off the gas pedal when we are speeding, or to check if the gun is really loaded. Even when the danger is only apparent, as is the case for spiders or open places for people with those kinds of phobias, the fear response still occurs appropriately to what is perceived as a danger.

Only in the past few years have doctors and scientists begun to speculate about the purpose of depression. It's about time. Why has it taken so long to initiate this important line of inquiry? Simply put, only recently have scientists begun to discard the notions that depression is a weakness, a lack of willpower, or a character flaw. Yet, the stigma tenaciously lives on in many minds and removes much of the incentive for this kind of scientific study.

The few scientists who are examining the purpose of depression are coming to believe it may be some kind of defense. Just as fear is a defense to danger, they theorize that depression may be a defense to what is futile. This view reflects mainstream psychologists' belief that our emotions are linked primarily to our perceptions of whether we are achieving our goals. The notion is probably an oversimplification, and probably only the first part of a long story to unfold, but whether we are satisfactorily attaining our goals has enormous power to determine our mood. As an example, these psychologists would point to a teen whose application to an Ivy League university is promptly rejected. With the attempt to achieve a prestigious education now frustrated, her brain might push her into a depression as a way to force her to consider whether her application was actually futile in the first place. Perhaps her SAT scores were too low, but she ignored that. Perhaps her transcripts and recommendations were solid, but she read them as glowing. If these were indeed true, and she continued to ignore the obvious facts, her next step, if she were not depressed, might be to continue the futile application process to another distinguished college. And the outcome would likely be the same—the rejection letter that always seems to come in the telltale thin envelope. Better for her, though, would be a forced pause to take stock. Was the goal realistic? Did I have the qualifications? Could I succeed at such a university if I were admitted? These psychologists say that failure at a marriage, failure on the job, or any kind of significant defeat might prompt depression in order to slow down, even shut down, our thinking. This has good purpose. The downtime protects us from making snap judgments, or from jumping right away to another bad marriage or overtaxing job.

Scientists are also hinting that there is more to depression than disengaging us from fruitless efforts. A depression, they say, signals a yielding in an unproductive or dangerous conflict with a superior, regulates how and where we invest our personal energies, and communicates to others a need for help. Because depression is so common, and because it has symptoms related to the experiences of most people, they say depression cannot be a flaw. It must be a defense, although still a poorly understood one. Only if the stigma gets beaten down will scientists and doctors turn in greater numbers to figuring out what the purposes of this dark and cryptic thing called depression could be.

That is not to say all depressions turn out to be useful. Depressions that are prolonged, accompanied by delusions, or result in suicide can hardly be considered productive. But the ruinous outcome of an extreme depression cannot discount the possible value of a mild or moderate depression. The same is true of pain and fear. The gnawing extreme pain of terminal cancer or the consuming fear of a panic attack are aberrations of otherwise useful brain responses. Even altruistic lymphocytes go awry. When they get confused, or when they go all out, they may attack tissues of the body that they call home. The result is often a disastrous autoimmune disease such as lupus. The truth is not easily found in the aberrations and the extremes.

Author Andrew Solomon looked for purpose in the three episodes of depression he suffered. He writes that "those of us who have survived stand to find something in it." He concludes that formerly depressed people often are more benevolent, have better judgment, and understand the value of intimacy. "It is a window onto truth," he says. Dr. Henry Emmons also takes a particularly humanistic view of depression. He has treated hundreds of college students for it, and so I asked his opinions about the possible utility of depression.

Q. *Do you think depression has a useful purpose?*

A. Some suffering is good for you. I don't advocate suffering. But, if it comes, it can bring gifts. Having to deal with something as severe as depression stops everything. It brings you to your knees. It is a cause for deeper reflection, not while you're depressed, of course, because it skews your thinking then, but later on. It is a stimulus to look harder.

Q. *Does a depressed person get a sharper eye for the truth?*

A. People who are mildly depressed probably have a more accurate grasp of reality. For people who start out more positive, it serves them well. For people who are negative, sometimes the truth is too much.

Q. *Does depression teach you about intimacy?*

A. Depression teaches people a lot about intimacy. In many ways, depression is a call to community and intimacy, because depression causes such a sense of isolation and loneliness. It makes people realize how important it is to have authentic relationships. And I emphasize *authentic.* Some depressed people discover the capacity for intimacy in themselves and offer it to others. Then, too, people around the depressed person get a chance to become more intimate than they were. They have a chance to express kindness, compassion, understanding, and patience—to become a healing presence. A great deal can be said for healing by responding in a loving way. It doesn't necessarily break through the consciousness of the depressed person, but it gives that person a lifeline, a tether.

Q. *That's all fine. But isn't depression a harsh teacher?*

A. For sure. Depression is a very harsh way to learn, but it is still an invitation to awaken to a fuller and more vital life than before. I wouldn't advocate anyone in the midst of their depression to take up the invitation at that time. The mind is too distracted. But they learn as they emerge from it. This is especially true of a milder depression in a young person. What happens to a teenager is the same thing that happens when a nonfatal heart attack happens to an adult. You take stock. You listen to whether your interior monologue sounds right. This can go a long way to prevent recurrences of the depression. Depression can also break through denial. Some teenagers need a harsh teacher to defeat the denial so they can listen to themselves and their family. They can finally face the fact that they're choosing something that contributes to this depression, and they need to change it.

Q. *Can such a harsh teacher worsen your character in the process?*

A. Depression is an awakening, a cause for transformation. It's an invitation to become something better than our previous self. We all have our own darknesses that existed before the depression. For example, if our beliefs are very cynical, the depression might reinforce the cynicism. What's important is that depressed people have a choice as to how they will respond to their depression. Although depression can't change character, it can overlay aspects of character. Sometimes people who were once vibrant, playful, and had a lot of joy in life don't recover from the depression with those qualities, so they interpret that they are a different person. I would interpret that outcome instead as aspects of the illness lingering on, not a change of character. Their goal ought to be to get back to that prior state.

Q. *Can such a harsh teacher worsen relationships?*

A. Depression can heal relationships, but not everyone has this experience. It forces those around the depressed person to figure out how to deal with the depression and enlarges them in the process. It forces loved ones to be more attentive to that person. Depression can cause a greater capacity for acceptance of other people's flaws, shortcomings, and suffering. There is a deepening of compassion and understanding for others. For some people, however, it reinforces the stigma. But for those who deal with it head-on, it breaks down the stigma and barriers. It can also force an entire family into counseling, and for the better. That one move heals lots of relationships.

Coda: Partnering Parents Reflect on the Outcome

After finishing all the interviews for this book, I concluded that parents of depressed teens might have put more effort into thinking about the purposes of depression than have the scientists so far. Moreover, parents' opinions have been forged in the fire. I've asked some of them to offer their insights as to how depression may have benefited their teen or themselves.

Choosing battles and choosing helpers. Michelle had a comorbid oppositional-defiant disorder. Besides being depressed, she was incorrigible, rebellious, and prone to saying hurtful things to her parents and sister. Frequent minor confrontations were often punctuated with major crises. Communication broke down. This is what her father said about how those awful high school years prompted his family to grow.

"That time was so bad that I could never wish anything like it on anyone. Michelle and I learned a lot from those times. Michelle learned that depression is such a miserable experience that she will do anything to avoid going back to it. She pays close attention to her emotions and to things which affect them for the worse. She's more watchful than the average person, and I think she'll stay emotionally on track better than the average person. She's also very sensitive to positive feedback. She was down so deep before, it gives her twice the lift now.

"I learned how to pick my battles with her better. Managing a child is always an evolution, and her depression helped my evolution along. We used to argue constantly. Many of the arguments weren't about really important things. Now that she is twenty, I don't manage her like when she was five, but I do have to micromanage her sometimes. I'm really careful that I pick only important issues. Last week she called me from college and said she was going to become a cocktail waitress at a bar near campus. I quietly told her what I thought and said she could ignore my advice and do whatever she wanted. I didn't make an issue out of it.

"[My wife] and I had lost so much rapport with Michelle that we had to search for others to help. We were surprised how it all turned out. Michelle always said the most hurtful things to her sister. But we recognized right away that she always paid real close attention to what her sister had to say. That's because she was five and a half years older, intelligent, and Michelle respected her. We asked [her sister] to coach Michelle despite the hurt, and she did. She really rose to the occasion. Michelle's grandfather, my father, was really helpful. He was eighty but still sharp. He came from the old school of believing that all you had to do was give a child love, and everything would turn out all right. After watching Michelle, he gave up on that belief. He even went out and bought a copy of *Reviving Ophelia* to understand Michelle better. I'm still amazed that an old man would push himself to think such new thoughts. He lived in Chicago but would call her every day. He would fly in to visit her often, and they could talk about her problems at the Barnes and Noble coffee shop for three hours. Sometimes they finished their conversations in tears. He died a year ago."

A fuller appreciation of joyfulness. *Matthew's self-esteem collapsed with the depression. He struggled to regain it and finally did so in a big way. Formerly depressed people say that they covet joyful times, appreciate them to the fullest, and never waste them. This is what his stepfather had to say about Matthew's epiphany.*

"He became terribly afraid of failing. It was always the hovering bug. He had big mood swings. He was exuberant for a day, but it didn't carry over to the next day. He was afraid of interpersonal relations, tests, jobs, even conversations. He had so many good things going on in his life, but he focused on the bad. Finally, something made him want to step out on the edge. We flew down to Tampa and drove down the coast to the Keys. We spent five days there acting very bohemian. We drank beer and smoked cigars. He saw a sign that said 'Sky Dive Key West.' He said, 'I want to do that.' Now, Matthew's afraid to get on a stepladder. He jumped out of an airplane at 10,200 feet. He always smiles when he shows the video. It was the start of him being positive. There were several other incidents like that. He transitioned. He got a girlfriend. He was having a great time."

Insights may come, but not until long after the depression is over. Chloe suffered several episodes of depression starting in high school. She is a vegetarian who pays unusually close attention to her body. She is a fine arts major and has had several exhibitions. Her mother says Chloe is only slowly finding purpose for her illness.

"Fear makes her sick. I know she can make herself sick this way. Two years ago she was overseas in Kenya living in a small village to do an art project. She was disorganized and worried. She didn't get going on the project. She was stressed-out. She wound up sick and sweating in bed for two days. She was convinced she had malaria, but her blood tests were negative. She got going on the project and then felt miraculously better. She is sure she created her depressions. She thinks she should take responsibility, but she doesn't understand her exact role. She always asks, 'Why did I torture myself like that?' That's the million-dollar question. Maybe with time. Maybe she has to wait a while and get some distance. Chloe's just starting now to learn about her depressions in the past. I'm worried she may not want to know the whole truth, because she says she is afraid the insights might set it off again. She's a big believer that illness is a way your body tries to teach you something. It will take a long time, but I think she will learn from all this."

Parents get another invitation to develop open-mindedness about their children. Jared was depressed and also had severe ADHD. He tried everyone's patience, was considered an unattractive teen, and suffered repeated painful rejections. Here is what his mother said.

"This morning on the radio some commentator was talking about embracing and loving your children no matter what they do. I have been disappointed with what Jared has done with his life. But I look at all the positives. He's a great kid. He doesn't do drugs or any of those bad things. You know the statistics for ADHD kids. He's a relative success. It's still tough for me. I cry in my room. I burst into sobs sometimes. I knew I wasn't going to make a big impact on his ultimate success in life. The depression has taught me a tolerance for my kids that I ordinarily wouldn't have.

A severe depression may benefit only the parents or other family members. After a prolonged depression with a devastating comorbid condition, Frank dropped out of college and committed suicide at home. Because of her devout faith, Frank's mother sees some benefit in this ultimate of tragedies for her family and acquaintances.

"My prayer from the day I tried desperately to breathe life back into Frank's lifeless body has been that God would bring good out of this tragedy. It's been a goal of mine now to reach out to others on this journey. I don't want anyone else to live through what I lived through. A friend of mine lives in another town forty-five minutes away. She lost her son nine months ago the same way I lost Frank. He hung himself. It was their only child. She became depressed and was hospitalized twice on a suicide watch. Today is her son's eighteenth birthday, and I will call her. We e-mail back and forth a lot, too. She's struggling. She goes to the cemetery a lot. She keeps asking me if I am normal. After going through your child's suicide, nothing is normal.

"I've made little cards with my name and Web site on them. I hand them out at my church. I tell people to have their neighbors call me. One woman did. Her sixteen-year-old son just shot himself in the woods behind her house. I've talked to her and her husband. I intend to remember his death date and his birthday.

"Last August, I walked in a suicide-prevention walk in Washington, D.C. It was sponsored by the American Foundation for Suicide Prevention [AFSP]. I walked twenty-six miles from sundown to sunrise with other parents and siblings who lost loved ones to suicide. There were also people who were suffering from depression and had considered suicide. It was a healing experience because I could talk to other mothers who had gone through this. After I got back, my husband and I decided to sponsor a golf tournament in Frank's honor. We will donate the proceeds to the AFSP. Depression is like cancer. It takes people's lives. I would invite anyone to log on to Frank's memorial Web site, www.hometown@aol.com/lleat15328.

"After Frank's death, I insisted that the whole family go to counseling. We each hurt so badly that it was hard to find the strength to hold the other up. It helped one of my daughters realize she needed to be on an antidepressant. We are closer. Every moment is precious now, and I don't want to waste them. I could lose my daughters and have to celebrate Christmas without them. I make an extra effort to make sure they're okay. I always tune in to their thoughts."

Confidence and empathy. *Dan is an emerging gay young man and experienced a particularly hellish depression coupled with vicious harassment at school. His father has been absent from the home for the past thirteen years. His mother has been his constant and ready confidante. She has this to say.*

"Dan can now stand up to rejection. It doesn't hurt so much because he doesn't consider every rejection as being personal. He wrote a paper for an English composition class a while back. He said I like to wear nice clothes. I like theater, and I like dance. I don't like pro sports. I'm still a normal kid. He used the word *normal*.

"Dan is very accepting of people who are diverse. He doesn't do it blindly. He still expects them to explain themselves. He's much more sensitive to kids who are depressed. There's one girl at school who tried to kill herself. She cuts herself, too. She's alienated everyone at school because she's cold and mean. Dan's the only one who's sticking by her. He says she needs him. He takes time to talk to her, invite her out to coffee, and make separate plans with her. [Some days] she won't move. She won't get out of bed. But she will be around for Dan. Even her mother calls and asks Dan for advice. All that came out of the pain of the depression.

"Our relationship would never have been so close. When you're spewing to your mother all the time how much you hurt, how you were sexually abused, how you might be gay, you can't help but get close. We're total soul mates, and in a healthy way. I know what he's going to say before he says it. He pretty much knows what I'm thinking. We have our blips, but we have no problems communicating. You know what he told his father about me on the phone a couple of weeks ago? He said I was his hero."

An affirmation that one is okay after all—and maybe better than okay. Eric had a debilitating depression and suffered a recurrence in college. His main issue was lack of self-esteem. Eric's mother is like any mother and can't bear to see her child suffer. She thinks he came out of it stronger.

"This whole depression thing was awful. I don't want to believe that anything good could come out of something like that. If there is one thing, it is that he came out of it feeling normal. He didn't go into it feeling normal. He had a chance to examine himself and to have loving parents help him with the examination. He's more self-assured now than I ever would have expected. I'm impressed with him."

Adversity Builds Resilience

It's a revered adage: "Adversity introduces us to ourselves." Having watched Eric's struggles, I think the adage applies best to depression. If it were up to me only, I would have chosen any way at all but the appalling adversity of depression for Eric to gain the precious self-knowledge that he did. I would never choose a teacher so depraved that he might take the learner's life in the process. At times in the late-night hours I still wonder whether the benefits were relatively trivial compared to the backbreaking travails of depression he endured. Depression is an expensive way to learn. Yet, I still consider whether the expense may be justified because the education is so efficient, precise, and quick. Eric got a doctorate in self-psychology during his sophomore year in high school. He had been handed a decade's worth of insights, maybe a lifetime's. Eric's lessons contained no useless details, no inconsequential material unworthy of a final exam. It was all important stuff. It was all useful stuff.

For depression, I think the adage ought to be expanded.

Adversity introduces us to new skills. As Eric emerged and recovered from the depression, I could see he was developing a new talent, a new defense, a new virtue—resilience. He was discarding negative thinking patterns and looking at the world through lenses less scratched. He is now more resilient when confronted with sadness, disappointment, or discouragement. He bounces back faster. Moreover, the coping skills he developed to tolerate the depression serve him well now in mitigating fear, tedium, unpleasant but necessary tasks, and the annoyances of disagreeable people. I am most impressed that he can prioritize his worries. Some things, an organic chemistry midterm, for example, are worth the fretting. Other things, he can now discriminate, ought to be no more upsetting than straw men or paper tigers.

Adversity introduces us to new outlooks. Eric learned to rejoice more in the good times. To be around him is more pleasurable because he celebrates the moment and takes it all in rather than just passively watching it go by like a parade float. He also became acutely aware of other people's burdens. For example, he could spot their vulnerabilities easier and make sure he didn't inadvertently bruise their psyches. He could spot their depression, too, even when others couldn't. In fact, he encouraged two students who lived in his college dormitory to seek out counseling and medication. They did, and they often remind Eric that they are grateful for his interest and concern. The adversity increased his loyalty to friends, especially those people who helped to pull him out of his depression. It also decreased his tolerance for those who are mean or hurtful, and he omits those people faster from his life.

Adversity makes us survivors. Being a survivor is a magnificent state. Depressed people who have fought their way back from hell get a certain confidence that may even border on mastery. Eric doesn't wear his confidence brashly with a medal. He wears it humbly, and with scars in place of the medals. He has gained a quiet inner peace and certainty that he can step lively and not be afraid of falling without being able to get up. I can hear the confidence in Eric's voice when he talks with college roommates about the usual problems of adolescence. I can hear it when he counsels his best friend on the phone, telling him to take charge and go confidently down the path of a solution. There is no time for whining, no time for hesitation, no reason to lay back and take some lumps, blindly hoping tomorrow will somehow be better. He knows, too, that if the depression returned, he would survive again, and likely beat it better. It's not that he is unafraid, but he knows he can put up a fierce and valiant battle.

Adversity clarifies for us what is important about our relationships. Eric saw proof that his acceptance by his family was not contingent on his being attractive, agreeable, or cool. He was a mess—and still dearly loved. He could trust that his vulnerabilities would not be ridiculed. Instead, my wife and I pointed out how they could be shored up, and even how they sometimes made him more endearing. Most of all, he realized his family was his safety net. When he was utterly defenseless, at least he could survive like a boy in a bubble, until he could reclaim his capacities.

Eric's adversity reconvinced me that the family must be the center of a teen's life. My wife and I made sure the family continued as an intellectual and emotional center. Eric had no doubt we were always available without notice for conversations and crying. We made the house the family's physical center by filling it with relatives, friends, and pleasurable activities. We even expanded the garden patch in back to advertise our claim that this safe place of high ground identifiably belonged to Eric and his family, and it would endure. I even recommitted myself to staying in good health and trying to live a bit longer. After all, Eric might suffer a recurrence, and I would have to be around to keep another watch. I might have to be a partner again. The center must hold.

Resources

Information on Depression and Related Disorders and Finding Professional Help

American Academy of Child and Adolescent Psychiatry
(202) 966-7300
www.aacap.org

American Association for Marriage and Family Therapy
(703) 838-9808
www.aamft.org

American Psychiatric Association
(703) 907-7300
www.psych.org

American Psychological Association
(800) 374-2721
www.apa.org

Anxiety Disorders Association of America (ADAA)
(240) 485-1001
www.adaa.org

Child & Adolescent Bipolar Foundation
(847) 256-8525
www.bpkids.org

Depression and Related Affective Disorders Association (DRADA)
(410) 583-2919
www.drada.org

The Jed Foundation
(212) 343-0016
www.jedfoundation.org

*National Alliance for the Mentally
Ill (NAMI)*
(800) 950-NAMI (6264)
www.nami.org

*National Depressive and Manic-
Depressive Association*
800-826-3632
www.ndmda.org

*National Institute of Mental Health
(NIMH)*
301-443-4513
www.nimh.nih.gov

*National Mental Health Associa-
tion (NMHA)*
800-969-NMHA (6642)
www.nmha.org

Help with Addictions and Family Dysfunctions

Al-Anon/Alateen
888-4AL-ANON
www.al-anon.alateen.org

Alcoholics Anonymous
(212) 870-3400
www.alcoholics-anonymous.org

Because I Love You
(310) 659-5289
www.becauseiloveyou.org

Narcotics Anonymous
(818) 773-9999
www.na.org

Parents Anonymous
(909) 621-6184
www.parentsanonymous.org

Index